Comments on **Acne** *– the 'at your* *from readers*

'Over all splendid – and I learnt a lot.'
Dr Stephen Kownacki, General Practitioner and
Secretary of the Primary Care Dermatology Society

'I will recommend it to my patients.'
Jane Watts, Dermatology Nurse Practitioner,
Department of Dermatology, King George Hospital, Essex

'Good tips and an interesting read.'
Polly Bealby, a teenager with personal experience of acne

ACNE

The 'at your fingertips' guide

Dr Tim Mitchell MBChB, DRCOG, DPD
General Practitioner, Montpelier Health Centre, Bristol; Founder Member and Secretary of the Primary Care Dermatology Society; Advisor to the Associate Parliamentary Group on Skin

and

Alison Dudley
Chief Executive of the Acne Support Group; Founder Member and Director of the Skin Care Campaign

CLASS PUBLISHING • LONDON

Printing history
First published 2002

The authors and publishers welcome feedback from the users of this book. Please contact the publishers.

**Class Publishing, Barb House,
Barb Mews, London, W6 7PA, UK
Telephone: 020 7371 2119 [International +4420]
Fax: 020 7371 2878
Email: post@class.co.uk
Website: www.class.co.uk**

The information presented in this book is accurate and current to the best of the authors' knowledge. The authors and publisher, however, make no guarantee as to, and assume no responsibility for, the correctness, sufficiency or completeness of such information or recommendation. The reader is advised to consult a doctor regarding all aspects of individual health care.

A CIP catalogue record for this book is available from the British Library

ISBN 1 85959 073 X

Edited by Gillian Clarke

Typeset by Martin Bristow

Cartoons by Jane Taylor

Diagrams by David Woodroffe

Indexed by Valerie Elliston

Printed and bound in Finland by WS Bookwell, Juva

Contents

Foreword

This book makes an outstanding contribution to the subject of acne. It is down-to-earth and packed with common sense, as you would expect from two such experienced and well-qualified authors as Alison Dudley, Chief Executive of the Acne Support Group and a founder member and Director of the Skin Care Campaign, and Dr Tim Mitchell, a GP at Montpelier Health Centre in Bristol with a special interest in dermatology.

It answers all the questions you may have on the subject of acne, giving straightforward answers to questions asked by people with acne and their families.

The question-and-answer format makes it very easy to dip into the book and find the answer to any question on acne – but then you will almost certainly find yourself reading on and discovering much more.

It is comprehensive, coherent and accessible – by far the best book I have seen on the subject.

In addition to being an invaluable guide for people with acne and those close to them, I believe it is an essential work of reference for health professionals, especially GPs and practice nurses, many of whom are taught too little about skin diseases.

Peter Lapsley
Chief Executive, Skin Care Campaign

Acknowledgements

We are very grateful to all the people who have helped in the production of this book. In particular, we thank the following for their advice and support:

Peter Lapsley, Chief Executive of the Skin Care Campaign

Dr Stephen Kownacki, GP and Secretary of the Primary Care Dermatology Society

Dr Ravi C Ratnavel, Consultant Dermatologist, The Paddocks Hospital, Princes Risborough

Jane Watts, Dermatology Nurse Practitioner, King George's Hospital, Newbury Park, Essex

Nuala Bealby, Acne Support Group

Carla Mitchell, beauty therapist

Dr Rod Tucker, pharmacist

Marie Cunningham, RGN, formerly with the Acne Support Group

and

Polly Bealby, a teenager with personal experience of acne

And, of course, our thanks go to everyone who contributed questions for us to answer.

Introduction

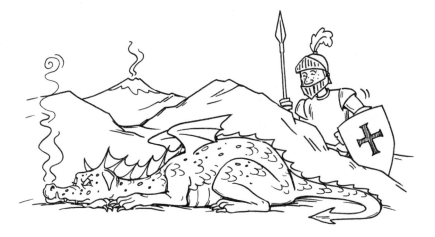

'There is a lot of it about.'

Nowhere is that saying more apt than in acne. More formally referred to as *acne vulgaris*, it is a skin disease that can affect almost all teenagers to some extent, with many people taking their 'spots' well into adult life. It is also becoming more common for some people to develop acne for the first time in their 20s and even 30s. A study in Germany in 2001, looking at a general population aged from 1 to 87, found that 26.8 per cent of people had acne. Looking just at teenagers the figure is more like 90 per cent. A few pimples and blackheads are very common after puberty but acne is certainly not a problem that can be dismissed as 'just teenage spots'. Sadly, however, it often is by family, friends and, worst of all, by some healthcare professionals. Many people with acne, therefore, get poor advice and information about acne and the treatments available, and fall victim to over-optimistic advertising campaigns while building up a collection of myths and misconceptions such as the following.

- It will always get better on its own.

- It is caused by not washing.

- It is caused by eating chips and chocolate.

- It is just a cosmetic problem.

- You can catch acne from someone.

- It's because you have too much sex.

All of these are **wrong** but commonly held beliefs and contribute to a lack of understanding of the problems caused by having acne, and this can worsen the psychological effect. Having acne is bad enough without being told that it is all your own fault because you eat the wrong things and don't wash!

As long ago as 1948 two American dermatologists, Sulzberger and Zaldems, remarked:

'There is no single disease which causes more psychic trauma, more maladjustment between parents and children, more general insecurity, feelings of inferiority and greater sums of psychic suffering than does acne vulgaris.'

You would have thought that we could have educated society a bit since then! Perhaps schools could provide some basic information about acne as part of their Personal Health and Social Education courses, and this is something the Acne Support Group is trying hard to promote. (The Acne Support Group is a registered UK charity that helps anyone affected by acne. As a dedicated acne charity, it provides unbiased, independent advice and support.) Even school nurses are often ignorant of the causes of and treatments for acne, not by choice but because it is not generally considered to be a priority. But it's far more likely that someone at school will need help for their acne than advice on head lice!

> *'When I did pluck up the courage to ask the school nurse about my spots, she told me that she didn't know what to suggest and asked if I had tried the spot cream advertised on telly last week.'*

Having a faceful of spots can close many of life's doors that are normally starting to open in adolescence – for example, to relationships and careers. Teenage years are very difficult and formative times as children emerge from the protective cocoon of family life to find their own individual identity and develop a sense of self-worth and self-esteem. Feeling upset by their appearance is the last thing they need, and seeking help from adults is not top of the agenda. Many of the myths and misconceptions are therefore made worse by being repeated among friends who, although well-meaning, often deter someone from starting treatment.

This book tries to answer the many questions that arise and should encourage you to seek help from a suitable health professional, be it pharmacist, nurse or doctor. The answers should give enough background knowledge to help you realise when you are not getting the attention and treatment you deserve and empower you to demand it.

As mentioned earlier, health professionals are often among those guilty of not taking acne seriously enough but this is a direct consequence of the inadequate teaching on skin diseases at medical and nursing schools. Various bodies such as the Primary Care Dermatology Society, the British Association of Dermatologists, the Acne Support Group and the Associate Parliamentary Group on Skin are trying to correct this, so, if you have problems, get them sorted out and then have a moan to your MP. You could also take this book along to your GP and encourage the practice to buy a copy!

This book is not just for people with acne. It is not just they who are affected – family and friends often have a tough time too! So learning a bit more should help them to be more supportive and understand the profound effect it can have.

*'I feel like I have had acne forever. My doctor was so
dismissive when I visited her, I came home and just burst
into tears. If my doctor can't help, what am I going to do?
Live like a pizza face forever?'*

Acne is also big business and uses up a lot of NHS resources.
Figures from 2001 showed that it accounted for well over
3 million consultations with GPs and some 50,000 referrals to
hospital-based dermatologists (skin specialists). This cost the
NHS more than £30 million but, in addition to that, people spent
tens of millions on over-the-counter preparations (no prescription needed) from pharmacies and cosmetics outlets, often after
TV advertising campaigns. These can be so optimistic that some
people get very disheartened when a spot-clearing cream doesn't
work for them. The ads seem to suggest success within hours,
when in real life treatments need 6–12 weeks to achieve a
significant effect. Failure at this early self-help stage can lead to a
feeling that if the 'TV cream' didn't work, nothing will. This makes
it very difficult to persuade people to use the right preparations
for the right length of time, resulting in further treatment failure,
demoralisation and, possibly, long-term scarring.

The cost of acne is not just to the individual affected and the
NHS. As with most long-term (chronic) diseases, it has an impact
on society from unemployment – 'spotism' can be a real problem
in interviews – and time taken off work. In 1984, when unemployment was running at 9.2 per cent for men and 8.2 per cent for
women, it was much higher for people with acne – 16.2 per cent
in men and 14.3 per cent in women. Acne varies in severity and
can be painful, and some treatments can cause inflammation for
a short time. The psychological impact can also be serious
enough to make life a misery. If you consider that acne can last
into the 20s, 30s and 40s, some people can spend much of their
working lives coping with it.

The psychological impact of acne is huge. Up to 70 per cent of
affected people feel a sense of shame and embarrassment, 63 per
cent have problems with anxiety (especially in social situations)
and 27 per cent suffer from depression. A recent survey of Acne
Support Group members revealed that 15 per cent of them had

sometimes felt suicidal as a direct result of having acne. All this is despite some very good and safe treatments that are readily available.

If this book gets all these messages across and encourages people to seek help, it will have succeeded. Remember that an appointment with a doctor for 'just a few spots' is not a trivial waste of time. Acne has just a profound effect on life, just as heart or lung diseases do, and is often easier to treat successfully. Read on and improve **your** quality of life.

> *'When I eventually saw an improvement in my acne (that I'd had for over five years), I was so delighted! Suddenly I realised I could get on with my life and stop checking in the mirror and feeling my face every five minutes. It's amazing what a good treatment can do, not only to your spots but to your whole life! Why didn't this happen five years ago?'*

1
What is acne?

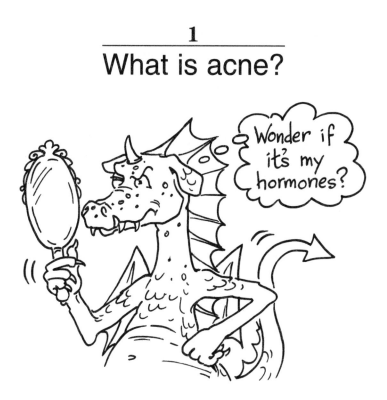

Introduction

*'Acne is just when you get a load of spots all over your face. You
probably need to have about 20 for it to be bad.'*

*'I think it is when you don't wash and your face gets all spotty
and horrible.'*

Acne is, in fact, the world's most common skin disease. You
know you have it when your skin develops blackheads, whiteheads, or red or yellow spots and becomes greasy. These are the
classic signs and it doesn't matter how many you have for your

doctor to confirm it as acne. Acne doesn't care who you are, what colour your skin is or how old you are. However, it is far more likely that, as you approach puberty, your skin will start to change enough to kick-start the 'acne process'. What most people don't know is that you don't always grow out of it: 15 per cent of women in their 40s are still troubled by acne, although for men is it less likely to carry on for so long.

It's a cruel fact that acne feels most at home on your face, but it can also crop up on your neck, back, chest or shoulders. This is because the oil-producing glands (the sebaceous glands) on your skin are most concentrated here.

There has been extensive research into acne, and dermato-logists blame four main factors in the skin:

- Firstly, the body seems to become extremely sensitive to the male hormones (the androgens) in the body. Women as well as men have male hormones but, because men have higher levels, they are often more affected. However, there do not have to be large amounts of these male hormones to get the oil-producing glands over-working, which makes them pump out more oil – called sebum.

- Secondly, these oil-producing glands have an opening into pores in the skin – small holes at the top of a tube or duct.

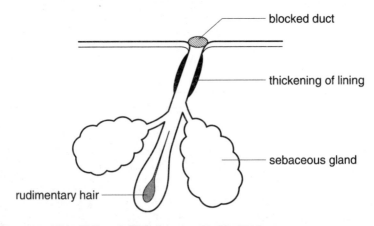

Figure 1 How acne forms

At the bottom of the duct lies a hair follicle – specialised cells that are capable of producing a hair. The gland opens about half-way up the duct, which is lined by cells just like the ones on the surface of the skin. If you are affected by acne, these cells tend to clump together when they die and are shed, and cause the duct to narrow.

- Thirdly, the combination of this narrowing and the excess sebum results in the blockage – the starting point for all types of acne. This creates a wonderful environment for the acne bacteria that normally live on the skin: they start to multiply, which can lead to infection and inflammation.

- Fourthly, this inflammation then wakes up the body's defence system, which sends white blood cells to fight the bacteria and repair the damage caused. These white blood cells make up the bulk of what we see as pus – yellow or greenish fluid produced by the body in response to inflammation; it contains lots of white cells that come out of the blood stream to attack the cause of the inflammation. But, if the blockage doesn't become infected, it will remain as a solid plug – or what we know as a blackhead.

Below we outline the types of spots you can get, so you can tell whether you have a mild, moderate or severe problem. They do not all have to be present for you to have acne. Just one type will still mean you have this condition, and there are effective treatments no matter how bad your problem is.

Comedones

These are the starting point of all acne. They begin as very small blockages in the pores. At this stage a blockage is referred to as a *microcomedone* – the comedone is too small to be seen. Microcomedones can progress to become larger comedones, or they can burst (rupture) internally, causing different types of spots. They burst because of the build-up of pressure and the damage that the inflammatory process does to the wall of the duct.

Whiteheads (closed comedones)

Some people think of whiteheads as a type of pus-like spots, but they are not. As the microcomedone gets larger, because swelling is building up behind the blockage, it becomes visible. If the initial blockage is quite deep in the pore, the opening onto the skin will remain closed; this causes the typical whitish lump that can be seen and felt on the surface.

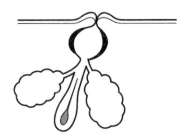

Figure 2 A closed comedone (whitehead)

Blackheads (open comedones)

These are clearly visible and very annoying because they look so dark and obvious. The blockage has occurred further up the duct, so its opening is widened and the contents are visible. If you were to dissect your skin, you would see the curly sebaceous gland – which is the escape route for oil – blocked full of a hard, yellow plug. This plug is a mixture of the sebum that has solidified and the dead lining cells that have been shed. Because these are like

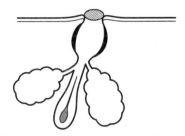

Figure 3 An open comedone (blackhead)

skin cells, they contain some of the pigment (melanin) that gives skin its colour. This pigment turns dark when it is exposed to air, so the 'black' in 'blackhead' is *not* dirt.

Inflamed spots

Comedones can stay quite happily in your skin for months, or even years, without changing. If they progress or burst (rupture), though, different kinds of spots result: papules, pustules, nodules and cysts.

Papules

If the comedones start to leak sebum into the surrounding tissue, this produces inflammation and a red spot results. Papules are less than 5mm across and have no pus visible. They could be called 'redheads', as they are otherwise like the whiteheads.

If your microcomedones rupture, you will produce papules without going through the whitehead and blackhead stage.

Pustules

A pustule is the typical pus spot or yellowhead. These occur when the bacteria present on the skin and in the duct start to

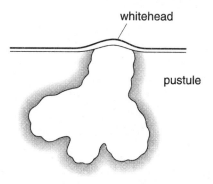

Figure 4 A papule/pustule

multiply. These bacteria are called *Propionibacterium acnes* (usually shortened to *P. acnes*). They prefer dark places with no air to breed. A blocked pore is ideal and soon there will be lots of bacteria producing more inflammation; this triggers the body's own defences as mentioned above, leading to a head of pus on a red swelling.

Nodules and cysts

Comedones, papules and pustules are nasty to look at and cause pain associated with the swelling and inflammation but will clear up without causing much scarring except in people with pigmented skin. (This is discussed further in Chapter 6, *The physical scars*.) The next two types of spot mentioned, however – nodules and cysts – can cause real and lasting damage.

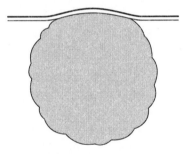

Figure 5 A nodule

Nodules

Nodules are solid spots; they are much bigger than papules and extend deeper into the skin. They are caused when a large comedone has ruptured, releasing lots of inflammatory contents (white cells and bacteria) into the surrounding skin. More inflammation and pus result, leading to more pain and swelling. The nodule extends deeper into the area that contains the skin's structural support. Damage here leads to the scarring.

Cysts

Unlike nodules, cysts are bags of liquid that is a mixture of pus and bacteria. Cysts usually occur only with nodules, often when two or three are close together. They are even more destructive than nodules to the structure of the skin but, luckily, are quite rare.

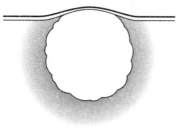

Figure 6 A cyst

Getting acne

I've started getting acne spots. How long do they last?

This depends on what type of spots they are and, even then, it can be very difficult to predict what will happen. Some spots will appear and then disappear during the course of a day but others will evolve more gradually through the various stages. Comedones can be very persistent if they don't get inflamed. Mildly inflamed spots will last 5–10 days before settling down, but can leave a flat red mark (macule) for several weeks. Nodules and cysts may last for weeks or months unless you get some treatment.

What is the difference between a whitehead and a yellow-head spot?

These two common terms describe quite different types of spot. A *whitehead* is a closed comedone where the pore is blocked and not open to the air. There is no inflammation (redness). A *yellow-head* suggests a spot with pus in it. The medical term is a 'pustule'. Whiteheads may become yellowheads if the blocked pore becomes infected.

My daughter is only 9 but she seems to have developed some blackheads around her nose. Can this be acne – like I had?

Girls seem to be starting puberty earlier and earlier, and many 9-year-olds have started to develop some hormone changes. Blackheads are one of the types of spots that occur in acne so, yes, this could well be the start of it. Almost all children will get some blackheads and other spots as they start and go through puberty, so your daughter will not necessarily get worse but this might depend on how bad your own acne was. We don't fully understand the role of genes in acne but there is some inherited factor that makes acne more likely in some families. If you had severe acne, it is worth starting a simple treatment approach to reduce the number of blackheads on your daughter's nose.

I am an identical twin and I have acne but my sister doesn't – weird or what? Can you explain why?

Answering questions like this is always difficult. We can't give you a reason why your twin doesn't have acne, because the precise cause and triggers are not fully understood. However, studies of twins have helped to work out that some genetic inheritance is involved, as identical twins tend to produce similar amounts of the skin grease called sebum. This is not the case for non-identical twins.

You don't say how old you are – it may be that your sister will go on to develop acne. She is certainly more likely to have acne than if she were not your twin.

I have been having problems with my skin for about two years. Can you tell me what the difference is between spots and acne? I think that to have acne you must have at least 20 spots but my mum thinks otherwise.

There is no real difference between spots and acne, assuming that the type of spots fits into the pattern we have described with blackheads, whiteheads, papules and pustules. What is most important is the effect the spots have on you and whether you have any of the more serious types of spot that might cause long-term scars. If you are upset by the appearance of your skin, it doesn't really matter how many spots you have – you have a problem that is worth seeking some treatment for.

Why am I the only one in my class who has spots? I heard it was very common but I don't think it is really.

The most important spots are the ones that you have, and you will be much more aware of them than anyone else. Other students might have spots that you can't see – on their back or chest – or they might be using some treatment or camouflaging make-up. Don't worry about them; just talk to your pharmacist or doctor if you are not already using some creams.

I get spots behind my ears. Is this still acne? They really hurt and they burst – disgusting.

It sounds as though you have had acne on the rest of your face from the way you ask if these spots are 'still acne'. They could be if you still have active acne elsewhere. There are also a number of other possibilities such as skin cysts or wens (sebaceous cysts – cysts filled with sebum) that are not connected with acne. You should see you doctor to let her or him have a look at them.

We've just discovered that my daughter is allergic to milk and cheese. Could this be the cause of her acne?

Unfortunately not. It would be good if things were that simple but studies have shown no link between diet and acne. As skin greasiness is increased in acne, it is very logical to think that cutting down on fats and oils in food would help – but it doesn't. Even if you are never be able to pinpoint the cause of her acne, it is sensible to get her started on a course of treatment.

My new boyfriend is really lovely, but he gets acne around his mouth and I don't want to kiss him in case I get it too. What can I do?

This is a common problem. Many people believe that acne is infectious and get more certain of this when antibiotics are used as a treatment. It is very important to realise that *P. acnes* is not passed from one person to another, so you cannot 'catch' it, not even by kissing him. But perhaps you can suggest that he see his doctor for treatment if he hasn't already done so?

A year or so ago I started to get spots on my forehead, which have crept down to my cheeks. In the last month, I started to get more on my chin. It seems to be spreading downwards – is this normal?

If this is what is happening to you, it is normal for you. It is always tempting to compare yourself with others and worry if you are not exactly the same. Don't worry that you have a different pattern of acne from your friends; it will still respond to treatment. The reason why it is travelling down your skin may be that there are different levels of sebum on the different parts of your face. Foreheads are often greasier than, or become greasy before, other parts of your skin so the acne spot will start there.

I am in my twenties and have noticed lots of small white lumps around my eyes. I don't really have greasy skin or other spots – could this be acne?

It doesn't sound as though you have acne. The little white lumps are probably *milia*. These are made up of dead skin cells and form small cysts just under the skin surface. They are common around the eyes and upper cheeks, and tend to occur when the skin is dry rather than greasy. Try using an exfoliant wash – this contains an abrasive substance, either natural like peach stones or synthetic like beads, to help remove the dead skin cells from the surface of the skin. Ask your pharmacist for an exfoliant wash and you should be able to keep them under control. If they don't clear, though, you could see your GP, especially if they are troubling you.

I get some lumps in my armpits which produce white gunk when I squeeze them. I have mild acne on my face but why the lumps under my arms?

It sounds as though you have two different problems, one of which is mild acne. The other is called *hidradenitis suppurativa*, which is a chronic inflammatory condition that affects the sweat glands in the armpits. It has some similarities with acne and can occur with it. You will probably have noticed a mixture of different spots – papules, pustules and nodules as with acne – but abscesses as well. An abscess can burst internally, leaving tracks of infection deep in the skin. Long-term antibiotics can help but sometimes surgery is required to clear the damaged tissue. You should see your GP to get the right treatment.

My dad has very bad scars and says he had something called acne congloba. What is this? I am very worried that I might get it.

The correct term is *acne conglobata* and it is, indeed, a very severe form of acne that can produce permanent scarring. It causes deep abscesses and severe damage to the skin. There are usually lots of blackheads over the face, neck, upper arms and trunk as far down as the buttocks. Nodules form where there are lots of comedones close together; they can ulcerate (break down the overlying skin), causing the scarring. It usually affects people aged between 18 and 40 who already have moderate or severe acne but the cause is not known. You must tell your GP about your dad, as this will make him or her more likely to keep a close eye on your acne.

My nose seems to be developing lots of burst blood vessels, redness and little spots. I'm nearly 40 and have never had spots. What can I do? I don't want to end up with a big red nose like a drunk!

It sounds as though you might have a condition called *rosacea*. This is common from about your age and is similar to acne in some ways. It used to be called acne rosacea to distinguish it from acne vulgaris but this caused confusion so the 'acne' bit was dropped. It consists of papules and pustules, but no comedones, and they have a much redder background colour. This is due to widening (dilating) of small blood vessels, which can look burst as you describe. Sometimes the tissue on the nose starts to grow and swell, causing an ugly appearance that has been linked with drinking too much alcohol. There is no link – acne is not the only condition with myths! Rosacea can be treated and you should see your doctor about it.

I seem to get acne just around my mouth. I can't see any blackheads but get lots of spots. The rest of my face is clear – why is this?

This is a pattern called *perioral dermatitis*. It just means 'skin inflammation around the mouth', and that gives a clue that the cause wasn't known when it was first described so Latin was used to make it sound better! It can happen in teenage girls and young women, and sometimes follows on from the inappropriate use of steroid creams but other causes are still not clear. You get papules and pustules but, as you have found, no comedones. If you have been using steroid creams, stopping will help but it often needs a course of antibiotics as well.

I'm black with tight curly hair and get lumps on the back of my neck. Is this acne?

If the rest of your skin is clear you probably have a condition that is quite common in black people. Tight curly hair can grow back into the skin and cause irritation. Firm lumps develop which look like raised scars (keloids). Its name is *acne keloidalis nuchae* – another descriptive term, as nuchae means 'on the neck'. Treatment can be difficult, so you should see your GP and perhaps ask for referral to a dermatologist. In the meantime don't have your hair cut close or shaved, as this can encourage the hairs to grow inwards.

A similar problem can occur on the face after shaving too closely. Lumps and spots develop and keep getting cut or grazed with the next shave.

'Grading' your acne

My doctor talked about my acne being 'moderate'. What does this mean?

To assess the severity of acne, it is graded into different levels. There are many different ways of grading acne, some very complex ones being designed for carefully assessed research into treatment. It is easiest to look at three or, perhaps, four degrees of acne:

- mild – mainly comedones with perhaps a few papules and pustules,

- moderate – papules and pustules,

- severe – deeper lesions, nodules and some cysts,

- very severe – many nodules and cysts with scarring.

These four grades take into account the numbers and types of lesions ('spots') as well as looking at scarring or pigmentation changes seen in darker skins. Each area of the body should be graded separately, and consideration should also be given to the degree of psychological impact. For example, if you have only mild acne but feel very upset by it, you should be considered as 'moderate' because this will affect which treatment is chosen for you.

An exception to the grading rule is in people with pigmented skin. Acne is one of the most common skin diseases in black people and can cause a lot of damage. There is always much more inflammation going on under the skin than would seem likely, so mild-looking acne in someone of Asian or African-Caribbean origin should be treated as if it were moderate.

Your doctor or nurse might also talk to you about grading so that you can check or compare how different treatments are working and how good (or otherwise) they are for you.

I hate my spots and have to cover them up when I go out. My doctor is no use as he says I only have mild acne. What can I do?

It can be very difficult to get doctors to understand how bad you feel your acne is but, if you always cover it up, there may not be much for the doctor to look at. It is worth following a few simple guidelines whenever you go to your doctor:

- Keep your hair away from your forehead so that any comedones and other acne lesions there are clearly seen. You could take some hairgrips with you and pin your hair back or up once you get to the surgery.

- If you are male and shaving, don't forget to shave on the day you see your doctor. Stubble can cover spots and make them difficult to see.

- Why not ask for the first appointment for the day? That way, you won't have to sit in a crowded waiting room, feeling self-conscious.

- If you really can't bear the thought of going without make-up, you must be prepared to remove it before consulting your doctor. In order to make a clear diagnosis, he will need to look closely at your skin. That is his job and he will have to look at far worse things than your skin, even if you can't imagine this! So take make-up remover with you and gently remove it just before going in to see your doctor.

Hormones and acne

My doctor told me I would grow out of my acne but I am now 15. If it is true that I will grow out of it, please can you tell me when?

Your acne will get better with time but no one can tell you when that will be and it is certainly not a reason to stop you getting treatment. Acne starts when hormone changes occur around and after puberty. These new levels of hormones stay the same for many years – until the menopause in women and longer for men. It is surprising that people do grow out of it but many more people seem to carry on having problems well into adult life. You need to deal with your acne as a 'now' thing so that when it does stop happening you won't be left with scars to remember it by.

Help! Every month, just before my period, I get spots around my chin. They don't even come to a head; they just sit there and hurt. Do I have acne?

Yes, you probably have. Acne is triggered by the skin's abnormal reaction to hormones, so the changing levels of hormones at the time of your period cause acne even though your skin doesn't react to different levels at other times of your cycle. This is a good example of needing to see your doctor when the spots appear, as there will be nothing to show if you have to wait a week for an appointment. It also illustrates how important it is for people with acne to be able to tell their own story about the pattern of spots and when they get them, rather than just being looked at quickly. Your history of getting spots at the times of your periods will suggest a different approach to treatment than if you had spots all the time. You could also think about taking a photo of yourself with spots to show the doctor how bad it can be.

I have heard that there might be a problem with my ovaries which is why I get acne. If that is the case, what is it and why do boys get acne?

You might have a condition called *polycystic ovaries*. This means that your ovaries have lots of fluid-filled lumps (cysts) on them. If this is the case, your ovaries won't be producing the right balance of hormones and, in particular, too much of the male hormone testosterone. You are then likely to have very bad acne, grow extra hair on your body and have light or no periods. In later life you could find it hard to get pregnant. It is very important to have tests for this condition; they include blood tests for the hormone levels and ultrasound scans of your ovaries.

This is one of the few times when tests are needed in acne. Your acne will need different and stronger treatment, and you might also be offered treatment for your ovaries. They are a lot bigger with all the cysts, so an operation to remove some of the cysts can lead to more normal levels of hormones.

Although girls also have some testosterone, boys' testes – the male equivalent of ovaries – normally produce high levels of this hormone, which is why they are often more affected.

2
What causes acne?

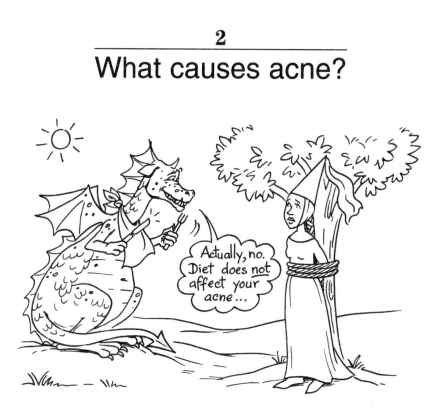

Introduction

As you saw in Chapter 1, almost all of us are going to have or have had some problems with facial spots, even if it is just a few blackheads.

Acne is a very common condition and we can describe in great detail what goes on in the skin to produce the various types of spot. What we don't know so much about is *why* it all happens. This applies to many medical conditions but research is always going on to try to improve our understanding. It is very frustrating not to have an answer to the question 'Why me?' but it would be wrong to pretend that there will ever be one simple answer.

Genetic factors certainly play a part but an acne gene has not yet been identified. Environmental factors are also important and there may be various triggers that set the whole process off. The control of sebum production is thought to be most important in causing acne, and more study of why some people respond differently to the same levels of hormones circulating in the blood will help us to understand this. The bacterium *P. acnes* was once thought to be the cause but we know now that it is not, though it is a very important part of the process. These bacteria live naturally in our skin, as do many others, and in normal circumstances cause us no problems at all.

In the past, doctors felt that a variety of other factors caused acne, including constipation! They also believed that diet was very important and advised a very plain diet avoiding soup, pastries and alcohol. We now know that this is not true but many people still search for a miracle cure, be it a special diet or a new cream. This is natural if you don't know enough about a subject. In this chapter you will find information that should help you avoid wasting money on 'quack' remedies that won't work.

Who gets acne, and why?

My doctor had a go at me about smoking and said it would make my acne worse. I think he is just using that as an excuse to try to get me to stop. Am I right?

Some scientific reports of surveys studying people with and without acne suggest that smoking cigarettes makes it more likely that you will develop acne or, if you already have it, make it worse. One such survey studied almost 900 people aged from 1 to 87 and found that almost double the number of smokers had acne. However, even this report concludes that, although there seemed to be an association between acne and smoking, there was little if any scientific evidence to prove this.

Nevertheless, smoking has its own risks and implications for your long-term health. If your acne might improve as a consequence of giving up smoking, why not use that as your motivation? Just think how good you'll feel in six months' time . . . and all the money you'll have saved!

If acne is caused by hormones from puberty, why does my baby brother have acne?

Newborn babies do sometimes get a form of acne called *infantile acne*. It relates to hormones but these have come from the mother while the baby was in the womb. Infantile acne usually appears in the first few weeks after birth and can persist for several months. Although pustules may be present, it is usually just comedones and papules on the cheeks and chin. Anything more severe or long-lasting than this needs investigation and treatment, as there are some conditions in which babies start to produce hormones.

It has been suggested that if you get acne as a baby, even if for only a short time, when you are older you might develop a more persistent type of acne. This could be an early warning to get treatment at the first sign of spots appearing in later years.

My forehead is all spotty but I don't have acne anywhere else. Why is this?

It is difficult to give you the right answer without seeing you but it is helpful to think about what is different about your forehead. Below are two likely reasons.

One problem can be your hairstyle. Ordinary hair across the forehead does not cause any problems but if you use greasy hair products, including hair waxes and gels, to keep your hair in a particular style it could cause acne. Greasy things can block up the pores and lead to the formation of comedones – we therefore call them 'comedogenic'. If this is your problem, stop using the grease and your acne should clear with or without one of the simple topical treatments. If your hair is naturally greasy, wash it as often a necessary with shampoo designed for greasy hair.

There is a type of acne called *pomade acne*, which is a direct result of using pomade hair products, more commonly used on African-Caribbean hair styles. If you wish to continue using these, you will need to keep it off your hair-line and wipe away the excess from the surrounding skin with a towel or damp cloth and keep your hands away from your face until you have washed them thoroughly.

Is it just me or are all burger restaurants staffed by kids with acne?

This is a bit of an urban myth but one that may have a little truth behind it. A hot sweaty face leads to more blocked pores and more acne. So the combination of heat and humidity in poorly ventilated kitchens where a lot of frying goes on and where everything gets a fine coating of grease can make acne worse. Also, these types of fast food outlets tend to employ students looking to boost their pocket money and therefore you have more teenagers – the classic age for developing acne. The worst cases of acne triggered by heat and humidity occur in soldiers on jungle training where the added friction from their packs (see the next question and answer) can cause an extensive and serious flare-up of acne.

I have heard that you can get a type of acne called 'handbag acne' where a handbag strap can cause you to get spots on your shoulders. Why would this happen, and would you have to already have acne to develop it on your shoulders?

Yes, this can happen. Guitarists can get this sort of problem from the guitar strap across the shoulder and back. The basic cause is pressure on that part of the body. This can happen in different situations; for example, violinists can get acne on their chin from the pressure on the violin chin rest. Tight headbands or a close-fitting motorcycle helmet could do this, too, and some soldiers can have similar problems from wearing heavy backpacks for long periods.

I am 29 and have just started to get spots. Is this the same as teenage acne?

Yes, it is but, although the same basic process is going on in your skin, it could have a different cause. Three questions need to be asked about acne appearing in someone over the age of 25:

- Is it a recurrence of acne that cleared up after adolescence?

- Is it a flare-up after settling down for some reason (e.g. being pregnant)?

- Is it a first presentation with no previous history of acne?

If it is truly a first for you, your doctor might want to do a little bit of investigation before treating you. 'Adult onset acne' could be due to drug treatment for other conditions, such as lithium for some types of mental ill health, epilepsy drugs, drugs used to treat TB and steroids. By 'steroids' we mean both those prescribed by doctors and the anabolic steroids used (illegally) by some athletes.

'Mechanical' causes should also be considered, as any constant friction or pressure on the skin can induce acne (see the earlier question about pressure causing acne). There are also some diseases that upset the balance of hormones in your body, leading to acne. Another possibility is that you might have just finished taking a long course of the contraceptive pill and your skin is now reacting to the changing hormones. This may settle in time, although you should still be able to get effective treatment to keep your skin under control.

A word about hormones

We have made much of the role of hormones in acne and it is worth saying a little bit more about them before answering more questions. The hormones that are important in acne are the sex hormones, which start being produced in large quantities from puberty. Androgens such as testosterone are the main male hormones, and progesterone and oestrogen are the female ones. It may seem strange that women produce some male hormones, but the oestrogen is made from testosterone by special cells in the ovaries. Not all of it is used, so some does pass into the blood stream and circulates round the body.

The female hormones can have a modifying effect on the action of the testosterone, which is why hormonal changes and treatments apply only to women. In general, progesterone will tend to make acne worse and oestrogen will make it better by making the skin less responsive to testosterone.

My daughter hasn't started her periods yet (she is 15) but has had spots for the past two years. I thought you had to have your periods before getting spots. Is this likely to improve once she starts her periods?

Starting periods is only one of the changes associated with puberty. Her levels of hormones have probably been rising for several years and will have had other effects on her body such as growth of breasts and sprouting hair in the pubic area.

She is probably normal but occasionally there are some problems with the mix of hormones that can produce bad acne and stop periods, so it may be worth discussing things with her doctor.

I've been told that there might be a problem with my ovaries and that is why I get acne. If this is so, what is it, and why do boys get acne?

You might have a condition called *polycystic ovaries*. To understand this condition you have to know a little bit about how the ovaries work. They contain specialised cells that produce eggs and the hormones to make the eggs mature ready for fertilisation and to maintain a pregnancy if conception occurs. Lots of eggs try to mature together and come up to the surface of the ovary in separate 'packages' (follicles) with the hormone-producing cells. Usually, one of the follicles becomes dominant and grows into a fluid-filled sac, or cyst, which then bursts to release the egg. This cyst can measure about 2cm before it bursts. If the egg is not fertilised, the whole process starts again.

Polycystic ovaries occur when twice as many follicles as normal start to grow each month and none of them emerges as the dominant one. We don't yet understand why this happens but the result is that many follicles survive to form cysts. These are smaller than the normal single cyst – 5–8mm – and gradually collect on the outer part of the ovary. 'Poly-' just means 'many', and all these extra cysts make the ovary twice its normal size.

As well as being larger, a polycystic ovary does not work as well. Slightly higher levels of testosterone are produced and it is not changed into oestrogen as efficiently. This leads to more testosterone getting into the blood stream and affecting your skin, to cause acne. Boys have a higher level of testosterone because it is their main hormone.

I have recently had a baby. She is now three months old and I am finding that my skin is breaking out more and more. It was fine when I was pregnant – this was the first time in ages that my skin seemed so clear – so imagine my disappointment that my acne is returning. Haven't my hormones changed for ever after having a baby?

During pregnancy your body produces higher levels of female hormones to make sure that it can support the changes needed for a healthy baby. This can sometimes make acne worse and sometimes better. Your hormones don't change for ever after having a baby, as they return to a normal state to make your body ready if you want to get pregnant again.

Another important cause might be your contraception. If you are breast-feeding and are also taking the pill, your doctor will have prescribed a pill that contains only progesterone instead of the usual 'combined' pill with oestrogen and progesterone. The usual (combined) pill isn't a good idea when breast-feeding because it can dry up your milk. The problem with progesterone-only pills – and this also applies to the contraceptive injections – is that they may make your acne worse.

I am fed up with getting spots before my periods. I had thought my skin was clearing, as I used to get spots all the time, but for a week every month it is as bad as ever.

You have a natural cycle of hormones during the month that make you ovulate (produce eggs) and then start to prepare the womb in case you get pregnant. The levels of the progesterone part of your hormones rise during the second half of your period and then drop back if you don't conceive (leading to a period). Progesterone makes your skin more sensitive to the testosterone that stimulates the production of sebum.

What doesn't cause acne

Since I decided to exclude meat and all dairy products from my diet, my skin has improved, with far fewer spots appearing. Would you still deny that there is a link between diet and acne?

It is always difficult to respond to this type of question. For you, the improvement is clear and you relate it to the change in diet. But it could be due to other factors, and the way for you to test this would be to start eating those foods again. If you then develop acne, you should stop the foods and see if it clears up again. If it does, you may well have a particular and individual sensitivity to those foods causing your acne. This would not apply to any of your friends.

An important thing to remember is that meat and dairy products contain a lot of essential nutrients and vitamins, and it can be very difficult to eat a balanced diet without them. Please ask for help from a dietitian to be sure you don't start developing new health problems. Any adjustments to your diet should be made gradually, as the gut can sometimes react badly to sudden changes.

My son refuses to wash properly and this is very upsetting as I am convinced his skin would be much better if he just washed properly. I have bought him all sorts of soaps and cleansers but he claims he doesn't need them, as he prefers to be 'natural'. He uses water and nothing else – that is, when he *does* wash!

There is nothing wrong with being 'natural', except that it doesn't always help to clear acne, especially in your son's case. Therefore if you buy a mild soap or cleanser of balanced pH (5.5), you may find that he is more inclined to try it. You can tell him that the 5.5 represents the naturalness of the soap on the acid-to-alkaline scale and therefore should be quite gentle while helping to remove some of the grease from his skin.

I am 15 and I must admit that I masturbate. This must sound silly but I find that, when I do this a lot, my skin seems worse. I even tried to stop for a while and my skin seemed to be better. Why is this? Does it really cause spots?

There is no direct link between masturbating – or any other sexual activity – and acne. Masturbating makes no difference to your hormones, so it cannot affect your acne that way. Indirectly, though, your spots might get worse if you get very hot and flushed from the exercise, as this can increase the chance of your pores getting blocked. If this is the case, wash your face with cool water afterwards and dry it gently.

My mate reckons that I have to use my own face towel when I stay over 'cause she is frightened of catching my zits. Is she a cow or is she cool?

There are good reasons not to share face towels but a fear of catching acne is not one of them. Acne skin is greasier and can have pustules that leak when you dry your face, so it would not be pleasant to share towels. She is right about using your own towel but for the wrong reason!

I have moved from the quiet countryside to a new job in Manchester. Since I moved I've noticed that my skin seems to be getting really bad – very greasy and with spots on my face that I never used to get. Is this just a coincidence or could it be that I am being affected by pollution?

If we assume that you are just as happy in yourself and have not started any new tablets or contraceptives that might affect your hormones, you might be being affected by the new environment or even the stress of a new job. But it is more likely to worsen any existing acne than to cause it outright. Pollution could irritate your skin and cause more skin shedding and blocked pores but this is fairly unlikely. Other things in your new environment could also have an effect. If your work is in a hot, humid place, this would be the likeliest cause.

I notice that, every time I go out clubbing with my mates, the next couple of days I get spots everywhere. Okay, I might take some Es but I don't reckon that would give me spots, because I drink lots of water which is meant to help the skin. Don't tell me to give up the drugs. They are just for fun and I only use them at the weekends.

There are far better reasons to give up the drugs than a possible effect on your skin. Street or 'recreational' drugs are not subject to any safety testing, so who knows what effect they could be having on you. New medicines are tested so rigorously that it takes years and tens of millions of pounds before they get approval for use in people. The clubbing is affecting your acne because you get all hot and sweaty and probably don't have a good wash to clear the sweat from your face before you crash out. The water you drink will neither help nor harm your skin but could cause you serious problems if you drink too much of it and take ecstasy tablets, as your brain could then swell and leave you in a coma.

Is acne an allergy to something? I am convinced our bodies try to tell us that we shouldn't be doing something, when they start to go wrong.

There is no evidence of allergy as a cause of acne. The *P. acnes* bacterium was once thought of as a cause rather than a factor in acne. Doctors felt this could be an allergy and tried to make vaccines against the bugs. Like a lot of other old beliefs, this was wrong and failed.

3

You and your doctor

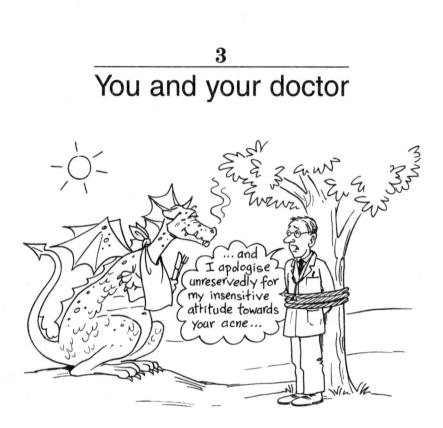

... and I apologise unreservedly for my insensitive attitude towards your acne ...

Introduction

GPs are busy people who have to deal with many and varied conditions every day. They are often overworked and often mis-understood. By learning how to get the best from your GP you should be able to work well together and avoid disappointment. There are positive steps you can take, and this chapter offers some simple pointers to help you.

Doctors try to do their best for their patients but some factors can contribute towards your feeling confused or an 'inconvenience' to an overworked family doctor. Below are some questions that are often asked.

Helping your doctor to help you

What is the secret to getting the best from my GP?

A vital part of getting the best from anybody is communication! Poor communication is often the cause of a breakdown in understanding between people, including doctors and their patients. Inadequate communication can lead to misdiagnosis or lack of urgent attention. This is especially the case for people when their emotional and social problems are not recognised or taken account of by a busy GP.

What should I tell my doctor?

GPs are not mind readers, so they need to be told about the physical and emotional aspects of their patients' illness or condition. To help your doctor assess your condition – including the emotional and social impact it has on your life – it may be worth making a note of your answers to the following questions.

- How long have you had your condition?
- What treatments have you already tried (over-the-counter products/other medication)?
- Where does the acne occur?
- Does it worsen at certain times, or as a reaction to stress or cosmetics, etc.?

Your responses to such points will help your doctor make a swift and accurate diagnosis. It could also save time for both of you. Letting your GP know you are taking your condition seriously will indicate that you are expecting a similar reaction from her or him.

Don't be afraid or embarrassed to describe a symptom or worry. Doctors have probably seen and heard it all before and will not feel awkward by what patients tell them. It is part of their everyday work.

Don't expect miracles. Be prepared to pursue different avenues – not every cure comes in pill form! Even if you are trying a particular type of medication, it may take time to find the right one and the right dose for you.

Ask questions if there are any aspects of your skin condition that you would like to know more about. Write down the questions as you think of them and take the list with you when you next visit your doctor. You don't get unless you ask!

Your GP should also take into consideration the following points, so be sure to mention them if any affect you, your family or your lifestyle:

- My condition depresses me sometimes/a lot of the time/all the time.

- I don't socialise because of my skin condition.

- I avoid school/college/work.

- Nobody appreciates how this condition affects me/my life/my family/relationships.

Once you have explained all aspects of your skin condition, your GP will probably start you on a course of medication that should clear, or at least control, your condition. However, there are still some questions you may need to ask to ensure you have realistic expectations.

- How do I take/apply the prescribed medication?

- How long will it be before I notice an improvement?

- Are there any side-effects I should expect?

- How long will the course of treatment last?

- How often should I return for follow-ups?

- If this treatment is not successful, what other treatments can I try?

- If the treatments don't seem to work, at what stage should I be referred to a dermatologist?

Try not to expect results too quickly. Treating acne successfully can take a long time, so don't give up. You will need to be patient and give the medication a chance to get to work on your condition. Make sure, too, that you understand the instructions so that you are using the medication properly. If you aren't clear about anything, ask your doctor or the pharmacist. And be sure to tell your doctor of any other medication you are taking, including vitamins and homoeopathic remedies.

I am 15 and don't want to go to see my doc because I'm really embarrassed about my skin. I also want to give up smoking, so I am going to ask about that first and then, if I can pluck up the courage, ask her about my skin. Even though I know I shouldn't smoke and she will probably have a go at me, I would rather put up with that than have to talk about my spots! Should I wait to see if she mentions them first?

You could do that and see how the consultation goes. She might ask you about any stress in your life that makes you feel like smoking and you could then talk about your spots. Doctors are now trained to look for 'hidden agendas', as many patients don't talk about their main concerns straight away. It is often easier to discuss something else until you feel relaxed enough to mention the big issue. But NHS consultations are fairly short, so try to give yourself enough time to discuss the real reason you're seeing your GP.

It is really frustrating that, when I make an appointment to see my doctor, it is always in at least a week's time. My spots seem to have cleared up a bit by then, and I feel he must think I'm making it all up! What can I do if I can't get an appointment to coincide with a flare-up?

The plan is that all GPs should be able to offer appointments within 48 hours. At present we don't feel that the Government is going to provide enough extra money for more doctors to make this possible very soon. Until then, discuss the problem with your doctor and show him some photographs taken when your skin is bad. You could find that your doctor is happy to see you more quickly and would be happy to have you fitted in as an extra next time. You must then calmly explain this to the receptionist and ask to be fitted in.

Some GP surgeries or health centres will also have a nurse with a special interest in skin disease – you might be able to see her or him more quickly.

My GP is totally brilliant, and really encouraged and supported me when I had my spots and helped to clear them up. Yet my friend saw the same doctor but didn't get the same sort of response. In fact, he didn't show much sympathy, just gave her a cream and hardly said anything. Isn't this a bit strange?

We are all human and don't get on in the same way with every-one. It could be down to a clash of personalities or an off day. At least she got the cream, though. Maybe she'll get more chat next time.

When we visit our doctor, it is important to remember that we are not going for sympathy but for treatments that should be effective and useful. Your friend probably felt discouraged because she knew of your experience and was expecting the same sympathetic response. Reassure her that it's the treatments that count. After all, it would be of little help if she had a very sympathetic doctor but was given no medication!

When you and your doctor have a problem

I'm really not happy with my doctor. What can I do?

The old *Patient's Charter* put in writing that you had the right to be referred to a consultant, acceptable to you, when your GP thought it necessary, and to be referred for a second opinion if you and your GP agreed this would be desirable. You should also be given a clear explanation of any treatment proposed, including any risks and alternatives, before you decided whether you would agree to the treatment. The replacement *Your Guide to the NHS* gives more general guidelines but the principles are the same.

If any of the above is refused and you are unhappy with the reasons, you should consider changing your doctor. If your doctor works single-handed or there is no other doctor in a group practice to whom you can transfer, you can approach another medical practice yourself and ask to be put on their books. Explain your reasons for wanting to change. You should not fear upsetting a 'medical mafia'. Most GPs will be sympathetic, as personality clashes do happen in doctor–patient relationships. If you cannot find another GP yourself, your local primary care organisation is obliged to find one for you unless you have been so unhappy that you have become violent. In this case you may find yourself having to see a doctor in a police station, so keep your cool, however unhappy you are!

If you want to make a formal complaint about your doctor's behaviour or the treatment you have received, you must send it in writing to your local primary care organisation within 13 weeks of the incident. Your local community health council will be able to advise you further, at no charge. (You will find both the primary care organisation and the community health council listed in your local phone book.)

It is always hoped that such drastic action can be avoided by ensuring that both parties have a clear understanding of one another's expectations. GPs cannot be expected to know every-thing about every disease, even common conditions such as acne. Likewise, patients should not be expected to have no wor-ries or emotional upsets or to follow instructions blindly, so speak up and share your problems with your GP. You never know – you could be pleasantly surprised!

If you want more information about what you can expect from the health service, ask NHS Direct (contact details in the *Useful addresses* appendix) to send you a copy of *Your Guide to the NHS*.

My doctor told me that I was lucky I didn't have a life-threatening disease, such as cancer. But the ironic thing is, my brother died of leukaemia only a few months ago and I found his comment to be so hurtful that I don't know what to do with myself. My acne bothers me a great deal. Should I report him?

Jumping straight in and reporting him would be just as bad as his comment. Ask to see him again to explain your feelings, or write things down if you don't feel able to face him. His comment about life-threatening illness was unjustified even without your brother's death but he may have felt he was making it in a light-hearted, jokey manner. Let him know you did not feel it was a joke and tell him about your brother, and ask him to take your acne seriously. If you don't get a useful reply, ask about the practice's complaints procedure to try to resolve the matter. All GPs have to have a pro-cedure for dealing with complaints, which usually clears the air. If you are still unhappy, though, you can take the matter further by complaining to the primary care organisation.

When I visited my doctor, she told me that it was no good my expecting her to examine me when I had make-up on. But, to be honest, how could I go there without my make-up on? I would have thought that, as a woman, she would have understood this. Anyway, why can't she see the skin? My make-up is hardly pan stick!

It can be difficult to make a proper assessment of your acne when you have make-up on. It doesn't have to be 'pan stick' to do a good job of covering up your spots. She could still have agreed to examine you using a strong light and just trying to count the number of spots you have. The fact that you feel the need to use make-up should also give her a clue as to how badly you feel about your acne.

You don't mention how the rest of the consultation went. The examination is only part of dealing with you and your acne, so your GP may have a good idea how to treat you after just talking to you. Try to see if there is a quiet time when you could see her without make-up, as it will help with picking the best treatment and checking on your response to it. Perhaps you could arrive at the surgery a bit early to give you time to remove the make-up before your GP sees you.

Each time I go into my doctor's room, he sighs, looks towards heaven and then says to me 'Oh, it's you again; what is it this time?' Really, I am not a pest, I just want my skin cleared up. But he makes me feel so guilty.

You and your doctor don't have a good relationship, so what has gone wrong? It may be that your doctor is not good at treating acne or doesn't realise the effect it is having on you. You, yourself, might also be part of the problem. Are you using the treatment in the right way and for long enough to give it a chance to work? It can be very frustrating for doctors if patients don't seem to have made sure that they have understood the instructions and carried them out fully. This may be because the instructions are not easy enough to understand or you have been given too much information to take in. Next time you see him, try to talk about your expectations from treatment – and his. If they are different, you both need to sort this out.

I want to see a dermatologist but my GP has said that it would be a waste of time as I would only be given a strong treatment that has terrible side-effects . . . and in any case the waiting list is so long that I would probably have got over my acne by the time I got an appointment. Is this right?

Sadly, there are long waiting lists to see a dermatologist, and this may be being made worse by the need to see anyone with possible skin cancer within two weeks of being referred by the GP. We probably need another 400 dermatologists around the country to tackle this problem. Although it is true that the only treatment dermatologists can prescribe that your GP cannot is a very strong one that has side-effects, they are not terrible. And it is not true that this is the only treatment you would get. Dermatologists have much more experience in using the common treatments in different doses or combinations, and often do not need to use the strongest treatment.

It is not a good idea to assume that you will get over your acne in any given time frame. You should be able to find out for yourself what the waiting time would be by ringing the hospital and asking to speak to the dermatologist's secretary.

I had an argument with my doctor about something not connected to acne but, when my daughter went to see him last week, he seemed really off. He said I was a pain and that he wasn't going to treat her skin because she was going to grow out of it soon and he wasn't prepared to prescribe her treatments. I am furious! What can I do?

Your doctor shouldn't talk to your daughter about you or allow a poor relationship with you to affect the way he deals with her. You should make a complaint to the doctor or the practice manager. The practice will have a system for dealing with complaints that will either sort it out to your satisfaction or show you how to take it further. This is the best way to approach any complaint, because it will allow some discussion of all the issues in a less formal setting than if you complained direct to the primary care organisation. Doctors often find it easier to say 'Sorry' in this situation as, once it goes outside the practice, they start to feel threatened and defensive.

If your GP is in a group practice, perhaps your daughter would like to see another doctor, at least for the time being?

I have been referred to an NHS dermatologist, and I feel that it was a complete waste of time. I was only in there five minutes, then she offered me a cream I had already taken and told me the acne would clear up. This is so unbelievable! I now want to see a dermatologist privately but don't know how to go about it. I looked through my phone directory, but there aren't any listed.

To see a doctor privately, you still need to be referred by your GP, who will have a list of local private dermatologists. Or you can contact the British Association of Dermatologists for a list of dermatologists who practise privately in your area.

Outside London, most private dermatologists also work for the NHS, so make sure you are not referred to the same person! It is also worth thinking about how you approach the consultation. Your GP may not have made a full list of all the treatments, so write them down yourself. Remember that dermatologists often ask you to try the same creams again but in different ways or for different lengths of time, as they can suddenly start to work, especially if you have had other treatments since you last used a particular cream.

I'm 25 and very fed up having spots all the time. My family doctor is usually really good but when I went to him yesterday, about my spots, he told me that he didn't see what the problem was and that he wouldn't give me any treatment until I have looked at my lifestyle. I think this is not very helpful – what should I have said?

Start positively and tell him that you usually find him helpful and really good! Then you can say that you are disappointed with his response on this occasion, as you are upset by your spots and have found out from this book (and the Acne Support Group) that there are no 'lifestyle' issues in acne. Ask if he is willing to treat you for this or whether one of his partners (unless he is single-handed) could see you for your skin while you remain with him for the other things he has obviously dealt with well in the past.

If he is single-handed, you will have to weigh up whether it might be worth changing doctors – remembering that he is good in other areas. Try listing those things that he may think affect your acne, such as diet, washing and so on, and show him how they have no effect at all. This will indicate to him that you have been willing to go some way towards doing as you have been asked while proving that lifestyle has no influence. You have then paved the way for your doctor to have no option but to give you treatment.

My acne is worse on my back than on my face, but of course I can hide that with clothes. I have been getting treatments (tablets and creams) from my GP. When I showed her my back last time, she nearly fell off her chair and exclaimed, without thinking about my feelings, 'Oh, goodness me, that is a mess' and referred me to a dermatologist. Why didn't she ask to look at my back before? I felt like a freak and really disgusted with myself.

Oh, dear! The problem started before this last consultation. It is very important to examine people with skin problems all over but this often doesn't happen. GPs don't get any formal training in dermatology so sometimes don't take a good history or examine patients fully enough. In a busy surgery it can be tempting to see the acne on your face and go straight into treatment. You may also be part of the problem if you didn't tell her that you had acne on your back as well. Her exclamation might have been because she realised that she had not been treating the whole of you, but she has done the right thing now in referring you.

My doctor had acne – I can see the scars on his face – yet when I went to see him about something other than my skin, he didn't even mention my face. I then read that doctors should be more positive in approaching patients about their skin, so I wonder why my doctor didn't mention it?

There could be all sorts of reasons, from pressure of work to seeing you as a confident person who didn't seem bothered by his skin. Doctors cannot be expected to guess what the problem is every time. If you are bothered by your skin, do mention it to him yourself.

When I asked my doctor for advice about my scarring, she had no idea at all what to say and got the receptionist to look through the *Yellow Pages* for a dermatologist or surgeon for private referral. I could have done this myself! As she is the professional, I would have thought she could have referred me to someone in the NHS.

The NHS is not good at treating scarring. This is really down to a lack of resources rather than a poor attitude on the part of doctors. Many of the treatments that can be used for scarring are only available privately, but your GP should be willing to refer you to a private dermatologist or plastic surgeon, rather than expecting you to pick a private clinic – which may not be as well regulated as you might like, and could cost you a lot more than it should. The British Association of Aesthetic Plastic Surgeons or the Outlook Disfigurement Support Unit at Frenchay Hospital (contact details in the *Useful addresses* appendix) can supply a list of respected plastic surgeons.

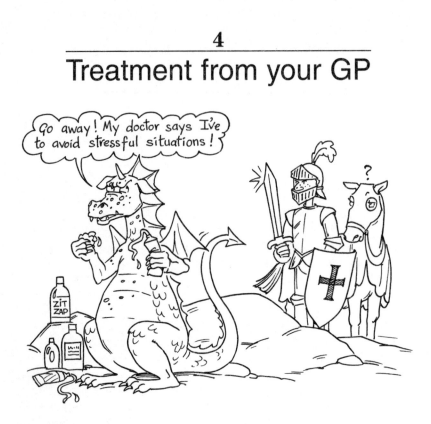

4
Treatment from your GP

Introduction

Although acne will eventually improve on its own, this can take many years and possibly leave your skin scarred. Most treatments do not cure acne but are very effective at stopping some of the problems. Treatment is aimed at:

- cutting down the length of time you have acne,

- reducing the inflammation in the skin and so preventing scarring,

- helping you feel better about yourself by reducing the psychological impact of acne.

It is therefore very important that your doctor or nurse knows how you feel about having acne. If you are very upset by it such that it limits your school or work or social life, you will need more or different treatment from that suggested by the basic grading of your acne on appearance alone. This is because grading is closely linked to treatment in the following way:

- Mild – usually only needs a treatment you apply to the skin (topical).

- Moderate – needs a topical treatment or two with a tablet (oral) treatment.

- Severe – needs the same as for moderate but with much closer supervision and more frequent visits to the doctor; .

- Very severe (luckily, rare) – needs urgent referral to hospital while taking the treatment as for severe acne.

As it is very common to feel frustrated about the time it takes for treatments to start working, it may be helpful to remember the Acne Support Group's simple 'two-month rule': it can take up to two months for you to see a result, so be patient. If, after using treatments as prescribed, you do not see any improvement in your skin, you should try another or return to your GP to discuss what might have gone wrong. If, however, you can see an improvement, you should keep using that treatment. There is no treatment that will completely erase your acne, so it is best to be realistic and look for an overall improvement rather than a total clearance.

The different types of treatment

Basically, there are two main types of treatment: those that you apply to your skin (topical) and tablets that you swallow (oral). The doctor may prescribe one or the other, or a combination, depending on the sort of acne you have and how you respond to the treatment.

Topical treatments

'I only slap on the cream when a spot appears, but I must admit my face gets red and angry in response! It also doesn't stop new spots cropping up.'

All too often you will feel the first tingle of a spot about to erupt and reach for the acne cream that may have been sitting in your drawer for the past year, expecting a miracle to occur instantly. Sadly, you will only be setting yourself up for disappointment. All acne treatments need time – and your patience – to work, and you will be expecting way too much from them if you slap on a pea-sized amount of cream onto one small spot! Below are some guidelines for treating your skin with creams, lotions or gels (the topical treatments):

- Apply cream sparingly to all areas usually affected by spots, even if there aren't any visible. Topical creams work below the surface to stop new spots forming.

- Don't think that putting more on will help it to work quicker. The chances are that it will cause a reaction in your skin and possibly make it look more inflamed.

- If any topical treatment leaves your skin dry and red, you can use an oil-free moisturiser on top without reducing the effect of the treatment. But wait for 15 minutes for the treatment to be absorbed into the skin before applying any moisturisers or make-up products. (To find an oil-free moisturiser, look for one that says it is suitable for oily skin types or spot-prone skin or is 'non-comedogenic' or is simply oil-free.)

- You can wear make-up over the top of treatments, but make sure that it is oil-free and 'acne-friendly' (this is how some skin-care and make-up products are labelled). Alternatively, look for make-up described as 'non-comedogenic'. As your skin is more likely to become dry and slightly flaky, creamy foundations may look a bit obvious. A light powder to match your skin tone might be more useful. Remove make-up thoroughly before applying your acne treatment at night.

Benzoyl peroxide

There are probably thousands of bathroom cabinets across the country that contain half-used tubes of benzoyl peroxide creams. All too often they are discarded because they can cause irritation to the skin, 'burning' off the top layer of skin and making it flake and peel. When you are trying to make your skin better, the last thing you want is for it to become more inflamed! But dermatologists and GPs agree that benzoyl peroxide is one of the most valuable ingredients around. It is useful at lowering the levels of bacteria on the skin and in the pores, and may therefore help to reduce comedones. If you start off using a low strength of benzoyl peroxide (2.5%), your skin is less likely to react angrily. By building up from once a day to twice a day, your skin will gradually become used to it. If you seem to be getting on well after two months, you can step up to the 5% strength. There is a new formulation (Brevoxyl) that some doctors recommend, which has a good record of causing less irritation: it comes in a 4% strength, which seems very effective and can avoid the need to start with a weak preparation and increase the strength.

As the name suggests (think artificial blonde!), benzoyl peroxide contains bleach. This works by releasing oxygen into the ducts and this kills the bacteria that are one of the causes of acne. The bacteria live in the pores because they don't like or need oxygen to live, so benzoyl peroxide is a very efficient killer and bacteria cannot become resistant to it. But the bleach will work on other things – clothes, towels and pillow cases – so you need to use old ones that won't matter if they get spoiled.

Azelaic acid

This preparation comes in cream form and acts in a similar way to benzoyl peroxide. It seems to be less irritant. At present it is available only on prescription from your doctor, but, as the trend is to allow more and more simple treatments to be available over the counter, it may soon be possible to buy it direct from a pharmacist/chemist shop.

Azelaic acid has a potential second use in that it can help to reduce the dark pigmentation that sometimes appears on the skin after the acne has cleared up.

Nicotinamide

This is derived from B vitamins and helps to fight bacteria while 'calming' the skin. It is available on special order from your pharmacist or on prescription from your doctor.

Antibiotics

The main topical antibiotics used are erythromycin and clindamycin. They are available in creams, lotions or gels, and need to be applied to all areas usually affected by acne. Erythromycin and clindamycin are the antibiotics most commonly used and they can be combined with zinc, benzoyl peroxide or another treatment called a retinoid (see later). Because antibiotics kill bacteria by using enzymes, bacteria can quickly adapt by evolving ways of blocking the enzymes and therefore becoming resistant to the antibiotics. This resistance of bacteria is now a common problem in finding an effective antibiotic treatment. Combining the antibiotic with benzoyl peroxide works well here: the disinfectant mops up the resistant bacteria. Even if you are not on a combined treatment, it can be worth using benzoyl peroxide for five days every four to six weeks or so to help prevent resistance developing and maximising the antibiotic's effect. Even if your GP doesn't prescribe this, you can buy it over the counter and start it yourself; at your next visit mention that you've done this, or perhaps even discuss it with your GP first.

Zinc – an ingredient in some products – is an interesting addition to topical medication. It comes combined with clindamycin in a product called Zindaclin. In Zineryt the zinc has been shown to reduce the development of bacterial resistance, improve the skin's healing process and delay the skin's absorption of erythromycin (the other main ingredient), thus keeping it where it is needed for longer. Zinc is part of the formulation of the product Zindaclin, rather than an addition, and also delays the absorption of the antibiotic.

The retinoid and antibiotic combination also works well, as it targets the comedones as well as the pustules.

Once the bacteria are resistant to a certain antibiotic, they will pass this resistance down the generations, and so that antibiotic should not be used again. It is worth remembering that it is the bacteria that are resistant, not you. This means that if you have a new infection, with a different bacterium, it should respond to that antibiotic. Doctors have many different types of antibiotic to choose from and some of the ones used in acne are not used for any other types of infection, which helps to control the problem of resistance.

Retinoids

These are substances either derived from vitamin A or made from a synthetic type of vitamin A. You may have heard of anti-ageing creams: these contain the same type of substance, although a beauty counter will only be able to sell a fairly diluted form of it. They act to prevent the formation of comedones, helping to remove the tiny blockages in the pores, so are ideal on their own if you just have the blackhead and whitehead type of acne. They can also be used in combination with benzoyl peroxide or an antibiotic, if necessary.

Retinoids are also used in tablet form but are then available only from hospital doctors. They have a lot more potential side-effects and need monitoring with blood tests, so only dermatologists are allowed to prescribe them – to people with either very severe acne or acne that is not responding to other prescribed treatments. They may also be prescribed if your skin is scarring or heavily scarred and in danger of getting worse.

Because retinoids increase the skin's sensitivity to the sun, you should use an oil-free sunscreen if you are taking this treatment.

Tablet treatments

Antibiotics

Antibiotics are the main form of tablet treatment and will be added in or replace treatments mentioned in the 'Topical treatments' section earlier in this chapter. Several different types are used, so if one doesn't work you can try another. Your doctor or nurse will explain the dosages and whether you need to avoiding taking milk or food near to the time you take the tablets (this can block the absorption of some tablets). As always, it is important to follow the instructions carefully to help stop the bacteria developing resistance to the antibiotic, and to be patient while waiting for the tablets to start working. You can, of course, use topical treatment as well as taking an antibiotic tablet, but, if you have been prescribed an antibiotic to use on your skin, it should be the same type – for example, erythromycin tablet with erythromycin cream. This will help prevent the bacteria from becoming resistant to two different antibiotics at once.

Hormones

The other type of tablet used for acne is a hormonal treatment called Dianette – the trade name of a drug called co-cyprindiol. It is designed to help reduce the effect of the male hormones, to decrease the excess oiliness of the skin (the main culprit in the acne process). Any woman taking this anti-acne tablet must make sure she doesn't become pregnant, because the active ingredient, cyproterone acetate, can damage the fetus. The tablet also contains oestrogen, which turns it into a contraceptive. If you are seeking acne treatment and contraception at the same time, you will be prescribed this to be supplied free of charge. As with any contraceptives, you should have regular check-ups with your doctor or nurse to keep an eye on your blood pressure and general health. Even if you do not require contraception, this can still be prescribed for treating acne but you will have to pay the prescription charge, unless you are exempt. (For more information about free prescriptions, see the section 'Costs of NHS prescriptions' in Chapter 9, *Sex, growing up and practical concerns*.)

Why are there different types of treatment?

Just as there are different types of spots, so there are different types of treatments. Some people may be affected more by the non-inflamed type of acne – the blackheads and whiteheads – whilst others may find that their skin is more prone to inflammation and pus-filled spots (papules and pustules). Some treatments are designed to help with both types, but more commonly there are two distinct categories of treatment that work best on one or the other type of acne.

As discussed in Chapter 1 (*What is acne?*), all acne spots start off as a tiny blockage in the pores, which, like a blocked pipe, will cause a build-up of pressure behind it. This is when inflammation and bacteria start to make the skin swell and look red, feel sore and start to produce pus. The first stage, the blocked pore stage, usually responds very well to creams and gels containing benzoyl peroxide or retinoids or salicylic acid. The inflamed stage generally needs antibiotics, usually taken by mouth, to help reduce the swelling and inflammation; then the use of retinoids may help stop further blockages. Some of the creams and lotions your doctor can prescribe contain a combination of two ingredients to help increase your chances of clearing your acne up faster.

It will always take some time to see results. No miracle cream or tablet has yet been invented to clear acne overnight – no matter what the TV ads may tell you! In order to get the maximum benefit from any of the treatments listed, you will need to:

- Read the instructions thoroughly and make sure you understand them. If you don't use your medication properly, you may reduce the chances of making your treatment work.

- Consider using your acne treatments as a routine in the same way you would clean your teeth: usually twice a day, with the direct aim of keeping bacteria at bay. Like cleaning your teeth, if you stop, it is likely that the bacteria will keep on doing their own thing, and your acne may return.

- Make sure any treatment you are given will fit into your particular lifestyle. For example, if you have acne on your back and you live alone, it is unlikely that a cream or gel will help because it will be difficult to apply.

How does my GP know which treatment is best for me?

A GP with the right sort of experience and training will be able to choose the right treatment for you based on your own story about your acne and by examining your skin. Your story will include how long you have had acne, how it affects you, any experience of acne in your family and what sort of treatment (if any) you have already tried. The examination will find out how severe your acne is and what type of lesions you have. Check the previous section to see how the treatment can vary with the type of lesions you have.

Using the treatments

How can a cream with antibiotics work? I thought you could only take antibiotics as tablets. How does it go into my skin?

Creams are used widely in treating many different skin diseases, because they are able to get through the layers of skin cells by dissolving in some of the natural oils that help bind the cells together. They therefore reach the part of the skin where acne occurs and have a 'local' effect. But cream is only suitable for mild to moderate acne. Tablet treatments will allow much more of the antibiotic to get into your body and skin, so higher concentrations can be reached.

I take antibiotics and they seem to be helping but it's very slow. Would it be better if I took more every day?

All acne treatments are slow to begin to have an effect but should then work reasonably quickly, so, if you have been using the antibiotics for more than two months, it may be worth thinking of additional treatments. This does not mean that you should decide to take more of the same, as this could be dangerous or simply unlikely to make a difference. Talk to your doctor and make sure you have a realistic expectation of how quickly your spots should be clearing.

My creams work well on the spots I can see but I keep getting new ones in other places. Do I need to start taking tablets?

Not necessarily. The acne process affects large areas of your skin and not just the spots you see at any one time. Check back to Chapter 1, *What is acne?*, and you will see that the early damage and blocking of the pores is under the skin and not visible. Always apply the cream to the whole area that can be affected, and you will prevent the spots at an early stage from ever becoming a problem as well as treating spots that you can see.

Does it matter when I use my creams?

It doesn't really matter, so, if there is a regular time that is convenient for you, try that. Just consider how you will manage some of the side-effects – such as bleaching of your clothing or bedlinen by benzoyl peroxide. An odd side-effect with topical tetracyclines is that they fluoresce (glow) under ultraviolet (UV) light – so putting them on just before going clubbing is not a great idea.

If you are in any doubt about when to apply your creams, discuss it with your pharmacist.

**The doctor has prescribed Dianette for my acne, but I am
only 15 and my mum will go mental if she thinks I am on
the pill. I don't even have a boyfriend, so why am I on a
contraceptive?**

Dianette is not just a contraceptive pill. It was actually designed
to treat acne, so the contraception is really a side-effect! Acne is
due to an over-sensitivity of your skin to normal levels of male-
type hormones called androgens. Even girls have a little bit of
these. Dianette contains a drug called cyproterone, which blocks
the action of androgens, and this is why it can be useful with
acne. It also contains oestrogen, one of the female hormones,
which adds to its effect and makes it a contraceptive. Only girls
can take it, because boys would have lots of problems if their naturally much higher levels of testosterone were blocked and they
were taking female hormones.

Share your concern with your mum so that she can understand
why you are taking something that also acts as a contraceptive. If
you have been getting lots of spots just before your periods, you
can tell her about the effect hormones have on your skin or get
her to read Chapter 2, *What causes acne?*.

**I have done really well with Dianette and want to keep
taking it. My doctor says I must stop now that my skin is
clear, as it has more of a risk than other contraceptive
pills. Can I insist on staying on it?**

This is a problem that lots of people with acne come up against.
Although Dianette is also a good contraceptive, it is designed to
treat acne and the manufacturers recommend that it is stopped
once it has worked. It may have a slightly higher risk of producing clots or raised blood pressure than some of the ordinary
contraceptive pills but is usually safe to continue with if you are
otherwise fit and well and don't smoke. You have to realise,
though, that this would be against the manufacturer's advice, and
your GP is quite right to suggest a change. A recently introduced
contraceptive pill called Yasmin contains a substance that seems
to act in much the same way that the anti-androgen bit of

Dianette does; it would make an excellent alternative if you are worried that your acne might recur if you stop taking the Dianette.

I have been using two creams on my face for about six weeks. At first I was really impressed, as my skin seemed to get better very quickly, but it soon got spotty again and isn't really much better. Why is this?

Each spot lasts only a few days before clearing and being replaced by new ones. We often find that new treatments work very well in the first few days and then seem to stop working. It is worth understanding that spots do not just appear on the surface. Because of the way they are caused by blocked pores and inflammation building up, there is always a new crop coming up through the skin. The treatment helps to clear up the ones on the surface faster than they would have gone, leaving a little gap during which you feel your skin has cleared. Remember this when the creams seem to have worked well and your skin remains clear – it is important to keep using them for a few weeks more to make sure that all the spots under the skin are also treated.

My doctor gave me Minocin, which seems to be working really well. How long should I be taking it for, and when do I know that it has worked?

Minocin MR is one brand of the antibiotic minocycline. It is a good one for acne, because you take it only once a day. It is good news that this treatment is effective on your acne but your questions are tricky ones to answer. In general, it can take about two months before antibiotics work 'really well' and perhaps three to six months before the skin looks clear. Once the skin is clear it is best to continue for a few weeks longer and then try stopping. Your acne may well stay clear for a while before gradually coming back but it is difficult to predict this.

Antibiotics are like all the other treatments that your GP can prescribe in that they do not cure acne. They just suppress it and prevent it from causing permanent scarring, in the hope that the condition will gradually stop as you get older. Because we don't know when your acne will stop naturally, we cannot say how long you will need treatment.

I can't seem to stop my skin looking like an oil-slick. I wash four or five times a day but it still gets really greasy. What can I do?

Greasiness is a problem for many people with acne and it can be as bad as you say. Sebum production is greater than normal in acne and some treatments are better at dealing with it than others. The retinoids, which are formed from vitamin A, are very good at dealing with greasiness; so is adapalene, a similar treatment. The creams, gels or lotions should help you a lot but if the problem persists it might be worth talking to your doctor about the much stronger tablet form of isotretinoin (Roaccutane). Because it is so much stronger, and needs careful monitoring, it is available only from hospital doctors.

I was on Dianette for three years and it was fantastic, but since I stopped it my skin has flared up. My doctor told me to go back on it but three months later it is still awful. I now feel desperate. What do you advise?

Think back to when you first started taking Dianette. It probably took a few months to work and this is the case even when you go back on it. You should talk to your GP and try an additional treatment as well for a couple of months to give the Dianette time to work. It might not work at all, which, unfortunately, is one of those things that we don't yet fully understand. Some treatments don't work the first time they are tried but then work later on, and we can't explain that either!

I was very happy taking my antibiotics for acne and they worked well. When I stopped, though, my acne flared up badly again and I'm as bad as ever. What else can I do?

You may need to go back on the antibiotics and take them for longer, or your GP might consider referring you to a dermatologist. The next chapter will tell you more about specialist treatment.

When my son used Zineryt, it worked really well. Then his acne came back about a year ago and the doctor prescribed it again. But this time it has had no effect – how come?

This is one of those things that we don't understand very well. The two main ingredients of Zineryt are erythromycin and zinc: it may be that the bacteria have built up a resistance to the antibiotic, but the zinc part of this combination should help to prevent that. We often see variations in how effective treatments are, some working well now although they didn't work before, and others that were effective don't work any more now.

You don't mention how bad your son's acne is. If it has come back in a more severe form, he will need to take antibiotics by mouth.

Associated problems

I often forget to take my tablets. Should I take more the next day to catch up? And how can I make myself remember?

It is best not to double up the next day, as higher doses of some tablets can cause more side-effects. If remembering your tablets is difficult because you have to take them two, three or even four times a day, talk to your doctor about this. Some doctors still prescribe tablets to be taken four times a day but they also work if taken twice a day – i.e. 2 tablets twice a day rather than 1 tablet four times a day. There are also one-a-day tablets that might suit you. Tricks to help you remember to take your tablets will vary from individual to individual but a couple of examples are:

- tape the packet to your toothpaste,

- in a prominent place, keep a photo of yourself with spots.

When I apply my acne cream, it stings and burns. It made my skin worse and I don't want to go to the doctor again. It's just a waste of time, so what can I do?

This is a common problem with many different types of topical treatments for acne. You must go back to your doctor and explain the problem and use another cream or the same cream in a different way. Topical treatments come in different strengths and in gel, cream and lotion form, so you will be able to try them until you find one that suits. For example, benzoyl peroxide can be quite irritant but a newer formulation of cream in a 4% strength seems to be tolerated much better. You could also try applying the cream less often. It is best to use a cream twice a day but at the start of treatment you can apply it just at night or even every other night, so that your skin gets used to it without becoming too red and irritated. It may also help to use an oil-free moisturiser about 15 minutes after applying the benzoyl peroxide to help reduce any dryness. A light moisturiser like this can be used as often as possible and will not make your acne worse.

My acne isn't that bad on my face but is pretty awful on my back. The last lot of treatments my doctor gave were creams and I just can't get them onto my back without making a mess. Also, I get through a tube in a couple of weeks. Am I doing something wrong?

You are not doing anything wrong. There may be a better way to apply the creams or you may need to use a different type of treatment. If your acne is 'pretty awful', it may mean that it would be better for you to try one of the tablet treatments, which would get round the problem completely. If not, or if you are not keen on tablets, you need to tell your doctor the problem and see what other creams you can use. Some creams or lotions are light enough to soak into the skin quickly so they are not messy and are good for putting on first thing in the morning. You might then be able to use another one at night and wear an old T-shirt if it is messy. The other thing to think about is whether you have anyone to put the creams on for you. Talk to your doctor or nurse and make sure they understand the practical difficulties you have. We doctors often forget about telling patients how to use creams and how much to put on, and often don't prescribe enough so it runs out and you end up feeling that you are a nuisance because you have to keep going back to the surgery. Find out the right amount and type of treatment and then get enough for three or four months!

Incidentally, the reason the acne is worse on your back is that there is more tissue there to be damaged by the inflammation in the deeper pores.

The cream my doctor prescribed for me rubbed off on my pillow and bleached it. My mum was cross at first but then she realised that it was the cream, and now she's worried that it might damage my skin.

Oh, dear! You must be using some form of benzoyl peroxide. The 'peroxide' bit gives the clue that it has some bleaching action. It will not harm your skin whatever colour it is to start with but it can affect the dyes in clothing and bedlinen. You will need to use the same pillowcase to avoid spoiling others or use some old ones where bleaching might not matter. You must also be very careful that it doesn't bleach any clothes you wear, especially if you pull them on and off over your head. There should be a warning on the package or insert that mentions bleaching but we always try to tell people of the risk. If you are using different creams it can help to use one in the morning and the other at night so that you can choose when to be careful about the one that is likely to cause bleaching.

My son has been given tetracycline tablets, which he has to take four times a day. He is not supposed to eat or drink milk for an hour before taking them. How are we supposed to manage?

This is a problem. Tetracyclines are one of the older types of antibiotics and still work very well if taken properly. This can be difficult, as you have discovered, because your son should not eat for at least half an hour after taking them either. The dose can sometimes be taken twice a day, which can make things easier, so talk to your doctor about this. If your son cannot cope with the restrictions, you should ask for a different type of antibiotic – there are ones that can be taken once or twice a day without the dietary restrictions. Tetracyclines are cheap but will be a waste of money if they are not taken correctly. It is much better to use a more expensive one if that means it will actually work!

My daughter just can't swallow tablets at all – they make her vomit. This is obviously a potentially big problem. I am worried because, when we talked to the doctor about getting rid of her acne, he said that she would need to take a course of tablets. Can they be crushed and taken with water? Or should we just wait and see if her acne clears up on its own?

If your doctor feels that your daughter needs a course of antibiotics, a wait-and-see policy might leave her with permanent scars. Although the tablets must be swallowed whole, she can certainly take them with water. Some of the antibiotics used in acne come in a liquid form as well. The most useful ones to try would be erythromycin or trimethoprim.

I get acne only when my period is due, about a week before it starts. But my doctor gave me a course of antibiotics to take for the whole month. Shouldn't I just take them when I get the spots? This would save me having to keep on taking them. I don't see a time when I won't get the spots coming up every month, so won't it mean that I will have to take the antibiotics forever?

You need to discuss this further with your doctor. There would be no point in taking antibiotics only when you get the spots, because they work to prevent the inflammation that causes the spots in the first place, so the long-term approach is correct. Something else to consider is that, if your spots are bad, you might be better off with a hormonal treatment; if they are only mild, a topical antibiotic might be better.

Can you set the record straight for me – does taking antibiotics long term cause future problems in other parts of the body? I am convinced it is responsible for my *Candida* infection.

In general, the antibiotics used in acne are very safe, even if taken long term. An exception is minocycline if it is taken in a higher dose than the usual 100mg or for longer than six months. Minocycline has been linked with some problems that affect the joints or cause different skin problems. This is rare, though.

There are a few niggly problems that can occur soon after starting on antibiotics. They don't just kill the bacteria on your face but can also kill off the 'good' bacteria that live in our gut and help our digestion. This can lead to problems with diarrhoea in the first week or so of treatment. In this situation the resistance of some bacteria is a great help, as very soon your body's 'good' bacteria will be resistant to the antibiotic and can carry on their good work. *Candida* is a yeast that commonly causes thrush. Low levels of yeast are also present in the body without doing any harm but can grow faster if the balance of yeasts and 'good' bacteria is disturbed. This can lead to thrush but, once treated, it should not be a recurring problem. Some people take drinks rich in the bacterium *Lactobacillus* to help the gut recover more quickly. You can get 'probiotic' supplements such as *Lactobacillus* from health food shops.

Another problem with antibiotics is that they interact with the contraceptive pill. They can stop it working but, once again, this is only a problem during the first few weeks of a long course. You will need to use additional precautions such as a condom for the first four weeks of antibiotic treatment.

My doctor offered to sort of 'lance' my big spots when I last saw her. I thought you shouldn't touch spots. I said no at the time, but these bigger spots keep coming up. Am I right to say no?

You are quite right if the spots you are getting are related to acne. Lancing is used to drain abscesses, more commonly known as boils when they occur in the skin. Follow the guidance in this book and you will be on the right track.

Things that don't work!

Is it true that dabbing toothpaste on a spot can help clear it up?

No. It is perhaps not surprising that you have heard this, as many people get so desperate that they will try anything. Asking people what they have tried produces some interesting answers! None of the following will work and might cause damage to your skin.

- Household disinfectants (even when diluted, they can still cause serious chemical burns).

- Cleaning powders.

- Dish-washing detergents.

- Industrial degreasing chemicals.

• Home facial saunas.

• Sticky tape left on the skin overnight and pulled off in the
  morning. Although this will remove dead skin cells and
  excess oil, it does not remove comedones and it might even
  cause more damage to your skin. And you might develop an
  allergy to the glue!

**I noticed that Sudocrem is meant to help acne. I dab it on
my spots but haven't really noticed an improvement in the
last few weeks. Should I carry on?**

Sudocrem, most commonly used to treat nappy rash, does claim
that it can help with acne. Our concern is that it could make it
worse, as it is a mixture of greases and other things that are
designed to treat nappy rash and bedsores. It is unlikely that it
will have any real benefit but, if you wish to try it, apply it regularly to only one small area of skin usually affected by acne. That
way you will be able to see if it is making your skin better – or,
more likely, worse!

**I read everywhere that you shouldn't sit in the sun for too
long because of skin cancer but my acne does seem to get
better in the sun. Should I try a sunbed?**

No. Many years ago, sunlight was recommended as a treatment
but times have changed and we now know more about skin cancer and premature ageing of the skin. The ultraviolet (UV) light
from sunbeds is not a safe way of getting a tan. Having a suntan
may help mask some of the inflammation in your skin but any tan
should be achieved slowly and safely. If you want to be out in the
sun and you are taking antibiotics or retinoids, talk to your doctor or pharmacist about this – some antibiotics make the skin
much more sensitive to the sun.

Your skin probably gets better for a short time because UV
light can reduce inflammation in the skin and make pores look
less prominent. This is short-lived, because, when the openings
of the pores close up, you are more likely to get blockages and

more comedones. Sunlight can also irritate your skin and cause peeling; the extra flakes of skin will also make pores block up more easily.

I have been given Papulex, which I'm told is derived from B vitamins. Can't I simply take more vitamin B to help my acne?

The cream Papulex does contain nicotinamide, which is vitamin B_3. It is thought to help stop the bacterium *P. acnes* from multiplying. There is no evidence, though, that taking a vitamin B supplement has the same effect.

If retinoid treatments are based on vitamin A, isn't it logical to just take a high dose of vitamin A instead?

Retinoids are derived either from natural vitamin A or a synthetic form of it. They are quite irritant, the tablet form in particular having lots of side-effects and needing blood tests to monitor its effect on your liver and the fat content of your blood. Vitamin A in large doses is also toxic and can damage the liver. Even small supplements can be a problem for children and pregnant women. Low-dose vitamin A has been tried as a treatment but needs much more research to see if it works.

Squeezing spots

I know that I'm not supposed to squeeze my spots but some of them really look horrible. Are there any spots that I *can* squeeze?

Although most doctors will tell you, quite sensibly, that squeezing spots should be avoided at any cost, there are still many people who find it difficult not to squeeze their skin. If you *are* going to squeeze or pick at your skin, you might wish to follow the simple rule introduced by the Acne Support Group, described below.

Traffic light guide to squeezing spots

If your spot is *red* (with no yellow head), **stop**. Do not be tempted to squeeze or pick at this kind of spot, as you are likely to cause more damage because there is nothing to squeeze out. This spot will probably hang around for a lot longer and may even scar if you try to squeeze it.

If your spot is *yellow*, it is **ready** and you may squeeze gently. The best way to do this is with clean fingers, and tissue to cover your fingertips:

1. First gently pull the skin apart, rather than squeeze and pinch the skin together. If the spot is ready, it will burst with gentle pulling apart. This should be all the pressure and force that is necessary. Any forced squeezing may then result in blood (which is *red* and therefore you should **stop**!).

2. Soak up the contents with the clean tissue and dab gently.

3. You may apply a small dab of tea tree oil (neat will be OK) directly to the spot, but do not apply too much as it could irritate the skin.

4. Now leave the spot alone!

If your spot is *green*, **go** to the doctor. (It is rare to have green spots, and very unlikely to be acne – we are just cheating because of comparing spots to traffic lights!)

Blackheads can be squeezed gently, but *whiteheads* should be left alone.

Squeezing at your skin will usually only add to your problems, so, ideally, leave your skin alone and let the treatment get to work on it.

The 'never, ever, do this' guide to squeezing spots

Some people have written to the Acne Support Group describing what they have used to try to help 'clear' their skin of spots or blackheads. ***Under no circumstances*** be tempted to use any of the following:

- tweezers
- needles
- pins
- Stanley knife
- nail scissors
- sandpaper (to help smooth the skin – not a good idea and very painful).

5
Specialist treatments

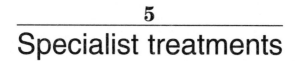

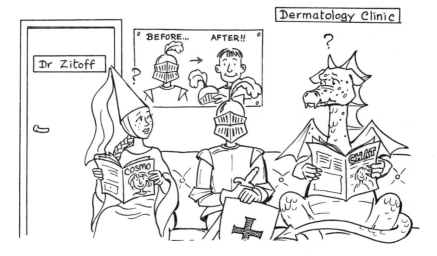

Introduction

Even if you use the standard treatments in the best possible way, your acne might need some tougher treatment or you could be left with scars. This chapter discusses:

- the most powerful treatment we have for acne – isotretinoin – which can be prescribed only by hospital specialists,

- some of the treatments available for dealing with unsightly cysts, and

- some of the treatments that are occasionally used for particular cases.

It is separate from the previous chapter on treatment, which deals with the standard treatments that well-trained GPs should be comfortable with prescribing. GPs sometimes need specialist help but getting to see a dermatologist is not as easy as it should be. There are not enough of them to go around: compared with other countries in Europe, we are very badly off with one for every 200,000 people. The next worst in Europe has one for every 80,000 and the best is one for every 20,000. The scarcity of dermatologists in the UK means that there will inevitably be a waiting list, so you must expect your GP to refer you early on if you seem to have severe acne. Waiting lists for people with acne are probably not helped by the need for dermatologists to see people with possible skin cancers within two weeks of referral.

Referral to a dermatologist

I swear I have tried every treatment going. I have had loads from my doctor but he says there is nothing else he can try. I have spent a fortune on treatments from the health food shop. So what's next?

It sounds as though you need to see a dermatologist – a doctor who deals only with skin disease. Assuming that you have tried everything suitable and for the right length of time to give it a chance to work, your GP may not be able to do any more in the way of treatment. So he should refer you to someone who can use different treatments or bring more expertise to bear. The following is a list of reasons for being referred to a dermatologist:

- Very severe acne.

- Poor response to antibiotics in severe acne.

- Rapid worsening of acne after a successful course of antibiotics.

- Severe psychological problems caused by the acne.

- Scarring.

Dermatologists have much more experience in using the different acne treatments and have one big advantage over GPs – they can prescribe isotretinoin, the tablet form of a retinoid.

Isotretinoin (Roaccutane)

I read in a women's magazine that isotretinoin can cure acne. Is it really that good?

It is a much-talked about treatment for acne and is seen by many as a cure. We need to be careful in promoting it as a cure because it doesn't work for everybody and there is nothing worse than building up your hopes only to let them down. Isotretinoin is certainly the only treatment we have at present that can switch off the driving forces behind acne – the excess production of sebum and the thickening of the ducts – that combine to cause blockage of the pores. Around 60 per cent of people treated with this drug will not need any more treatment but it isn't enough to help everybody.

If isotretinoin is so good, why can't everyone use it?

Like many good treatments in medicine, it causes side-effects that are well known and can be very troublesome. Often these problems will outweigh the potential benefit, especially if your acne is mild to moderate and is likely to respond to treatments with fewer side-effects.

The common side-effects are extreme dryness of the skin and soft internal surfaces (mucous membranes) such as inside the lips, eyelids and vagina. If you play a lot of sport you might be troubled by muscle and joint pains. It also can make your acne worse for up to eight weeks after starting it, which comes as a huge disappointment if you haven't been warned.

If the doctor decides that I should have isotretinoin, how long would I have to take it?

The average course is four months at a daily dose of 1mg per kilogram of your weight. Sometimes a lower dose is used to start with to try to prevent the drug's initial worsening effect on your acne – causing a flare-up anywhere between two and six weeks into treatment – so the whole course could last up to six months.

I am 22 and have had mild acne for about eight years, and I've tried loads of antibiotics and Dianette and acupuncture. A friend has heard about Roaccutane – how do I get hold of it? My friend says you can get it via the internet.

Roaccutane is the brand name for isotretinoin, a tablet form of the retinoids you can use as topical treatments. In the UK it is available only through dermatologists, because it has quite a few side-effects and you will need some blood tests before and during treatment. Because of the side-effects it is not usually used for mild acne. Do not buy it via the internet, as taking it in the wrong way or dose could cause you harm. It is also quite expensive: £400–£500 for an average course.

My friend went to a great dermatologist who told her that she could use Roaccutane on a two week on two week off basis, ongoing. This really seems to have helped her. My acne is as bad as hers was, but my doctor told me that this way of treating acne is dangerous because it uses the drug 'off licence'. What does that mean? Should my friend see another dermatologist for another opinion?

One of the ways that medical treatment improves is by trying different ways of using approved drugs. The licence for a drug is issued for certain conditions in specific dosages that have been tested in proper research trials and found to be safe and effective. The company marketing the drug can promote only this particular way of using it but doctors can try other dosage regimens that could be just as successful. This is what 'off licence' means. Your doctor is not right to say that it is dangerous, especially if it's used in the on-and-off way you've described. Some people use it for just one week a month, as for them this produces the benefits while keeping side-effects to a level that they can cope with. Your friend's dermatologist is good and is willing to be flexible with the treatment to get the best out of it for each patient.

I hate needles! Why do I have to have blood tests before and during isotretinoin treatment?

Blood tests are a requirement of the licence to use the drug (explained in the previous answer), and should not be ignored. The drug can raise the levels of liver enzymes that get through to the blood, suggesting damage to the liver, and of fat (e.g. cholesterol) in the blood. If there were a problem before starting the treatment, this could lead to extra side-effects, so your blood is tested beforehand to check this. Even if the first test is normal, it is sensible to test again during the treatment in case you are over-sensitive to the drug. In practice, liver or cholesterol problems are very rare.

The dermatologist told me to cut down my drinking before he would give me isotretinoin. Why is this?

This is because of isotretinoin's potential effect on the liver. It may be that your initial blood tests showed some damage to the liver from your drinking, and it would not be safe to add a drug that might worsen this. If you can cut down or stop, your liver should get back to normal in a few months.

I have been prescribed isotretinoin (Roaccutane) but have high cholesterol. Will this affect how the treatment will work?

No, high cholesterol will not affect how the drug will work. Cholesterol does tend to rise during the treatment but quickly settles back down to pre-treatment levels once you stop. You should still be able to have the treatment but will need more frequent blood tests to monitor your cholesterol. A higher level for the four months of treatment will not do you any harm.

I desperately want to take isotretinoin but my acne is so bad that I hate the thought of it getting worse. Is there anything I can do to stop the flare-up?

It is a shock to people when they hear that their spots will get worse when they start taking isotretinoin. But look at it as a way of clearing your acne by rushing through all the spots that are already forming in your skin. You might be able to lessen the effect by starting at a much lower dose and gradually building it up.

Another possibility is to take a steroid by mouth in the first few weeks. Steroids are anti-inflammatory drugs and can prevent the flare-up. They, too, can have side-effects so are not used routinely – especially as one of the side-effects of taking steroids for a long time is to cause acne! This won't be a problem in the short term, though, especially as you will be using isotretinoin as well. These steroids are different from the ones athletes get into trouble for taking, and will not cause you to grow big muscles.

I thought isotretinoin was working well but it hasn't quite cleared my acne. Can't I just take it for a bit longer?

You may be able to take more but it depends a bit on the total dose you have taken. The drug continues working after you finish the course, so it may be worth waiting a few weeks for the final result. Any remaining acne might respond well to a simpler treatment rather than your going back on isotretinoin and enduring all the side-effects again. Discuss it with your doctor.

The dermatologist was right – my acne cleared completely after the course of tablets. But I have been off it for three months and I think it is starting to come back a bit. Should I take another course?

Isotretinoin is reported as clearing up acne completely in up to 70 per cent of cases. But the reports seem to judge success by people not needing any more treatment by mouth. This leaves a lot of people who must have minor recurrences that respond to topical treatments. If acne starts to return after a course of isotretinoin, it should be treated as if it was occurring for the first time. A major difference in your recurrence should be an absence of comedones, as these are treated very effectively by the retinoid.

Your doctor should now start you off with a topical treatment such as benzoyl peroxide, in cream form if your skin is still a bit dry after the isotretinoin, or an antibiotic lotion. If these do not help and antibiotics by mouth don't either, you may well need another course of isotretinoin. It is always worth trying the simpler treatments first, though, even if they didn't work for you the first time around. Your skin is changed after the isotretinoin and any resistant bacteria will have been killed off, so the treatments will have a better chance of working.

I read in a newspaper that a teenager committed suicide because he was taking isotretinoin. Is this a side-effect the doctors don't tell you about?

Whenever isotretinoin is being considered, the doctor will discuss the side-effects with you, and you should be given a copy of the information leaflet provided by the drug company.

Over the past few years there has been growing concern about isotretinoin being able to make depression worse, and there have been tragedies where young people have committed suicide while taking the drug. It is very difficult to pin the blame on the isotretinoin, as many people feel depressed and contemplate suicide just because they have acne. What may happen in some cases is that a tendency to become depressed is made worse by having severe acne and taking isotretinoin. In the first few weeks of treatment the acne tends to get worse and this can be desperately disappointing. The drug may make mood swings more likely, so, if someone's mood swings down when they are already feeling very low, this can lead to the tragedy of suicide. People with a history of depression will need careful support if they are thought to need isotretinoin. They will need to have a friend or relative who can act as a 'buddy' – someone who sees them every day and who is there to pick up any warning signs of worsening depression or a downturn in mood. The doctor can then be alerted so that extra support and treatment is provided.

Why did the dermatologist ask me if I might get pregnant? I thought he was being a bit nosy.

He is not being nosy at all. It sounds as if you might need treatment with isotretinoin. This drug and pregnancy would be a recipe for disaster, as the growing fetus would be seriously damaged. To prevent any horrible mistakes, you will need to read and sign a form that says you understand why you must not get pregnant, that you will use a reliable form of contraception and will have a negative pregnancy test before you start treatment.

Reliable contraception is defined as a pill or the coil; condoms or caps can be forgotten, so they do not count! If you are on Dianette, you could continue to take this – it contains oestrogen, one of the female hormones, which makes it a contraceptive as well. If you are not sexually active and not likely to be so during the treatment and for six weeks afterwards, this is also accepted as a reliable form of contraception. The six-week gap after finishing treatment allows for all of the drug to be washed out of your system. This effect on unborn babies is the main reason why the company that manufactures the drug has requested that it be available only from dermatologists.

Other treatments

I am going to a big family wedding in 10 days and a big cyst has come up on my face. I just know it will still be there on the day. Can I do anything to get rid of it?

Some doctors are experienced at injecting cysts like this with a steroid. It must be done by a doctor with this experience, as it can cause permanent damage to the skin if the correct technique and strength of steroid are not used. If your own GP has no such experience, ask whether anyone else in the practice could do it. If not, or if your GP works single-handed, you would have to see a dermatologist, but even going privately you might have trouble getting an appointment in time. It is likely, though, that the cyst will have calmed down in time for the wedding. The moral here is that, if you are prone to acne, make sure that it is under control in advance of any special occasion.

My acne is much better than it used to be but I still have some hard lumps on my cheeks. Can I have them cut out?

You could, but it would not be a good idea because you would end up with ugly scars to replace what are probably old cysts. These can be treated with liquid nitrogen, which is very cold. It is most often used to treat warts or verrucas and many GPs have access to it in their surgeries; if your GP is not happy to freeze your cysts, you should ask for referral to a dermatologist.

I have heard about some lamps that treat acne. Do they work?

A mixture of red–blue light used in a controlled way has had some effect on inflammation and in reducing the number of acne spots. One trial of the technique involved treating the skin for 15 minutes three times a day for 12 weeks. It produced reasonable results in making inflammatory spots 75 per cent better but had no proven effect on comedones. It probably works by a combination of antibacterial and anti-inflammatory action. If you worked this hard at any of the more standard treatments, you would probably get as good if not better results. It also seems that the acne comes back once you stop the light treatment.

I don't want to take isotretinoin because I'm too scared of the side-effects. Is there anything else the dermatologist can offer me?

The dermatologist can try some of the standard treatments in different doses or combinations. The most common trick is to use higher doses of antibiotics. Both minocycline and trimethoprim can work well in higher doses than GPs are used to using. There shouldn't be any problems with the trimethoprim but the minocycline may cause some side-effects. In the higher doses of 200mg a day rather than 100mg it can cause unsightly blue-black pigment to be laid down in the skin. It is also associated with some serious conditions that can lead to liver damage or arthritis. As long as you are properly supervised and have regular blood tests, these side-effects can be prevented by stopping the drug if the dermatologist tells you to.

My acne seems to be made worse by my monthly periods so I wanted to try the hormone treatment. My doctor says it wouldn't be very safe because of problems with blood clotting. Is there nothing I can try?

It is the oestrogen part of the usual hormonal treatment that would cause you problems. There is a slightly increased risk of blood clots in some people taking hormones, and it can rise if there is a personal or close family history of clots. The anti-androgen part of the treatment is not suitable to take on its own but some dermatologists prescribe another drug that can have the same effect. Called spironolactone, it blocks the action of testosterone. It is worth trying but needs to be started at a low dose and increased slowly in case it produces side-effects such as menstrual irregularities, breast tenderness or fatigue. It also needs some blood tests to check on possible changes in some of the salts (sodium and potassium) in the blood but these rarely cause any problems.

6
The physical scars

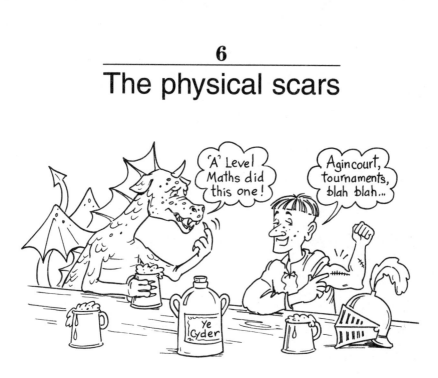

Introduction

As if having acne isn't bad enough, you can be left with a permanent reminder in the way of scars from the damage to the important structures deep in the skin. Before discussing these, it is worth mentioning some marks that could be regarded as scars but are not due to the same destructive processes. They are visible but should improve with time. The first of these 'scars' appears as red flat marks where spots used to be. Called macules, they are the last sign of the inflammation in the skin and can last for up to six months. The other 'scar' is the brown discoloration where the acne used to be – called *post-inflammatory hyper-pigmentation*. A result of the inflammatory process stimulating the pigment cells in the skin, it is more common the darker your skin is and can last for up to 18 months.

True scars are longer lasting and are a result of both the injury to the skin caused by the acne and the way the body tries to repair the damage. Some people will scar much more easily than others. The process is not well understood but it most often happens with severe acne nodules and cysts.

Scars can be looked at under two headings: extra skin tissue and loss of normal skin tissue.

Extra skin tissue (raised scars)

These are called *keloid* or *hypertrophic* scars ('hypertrophic' means enlargement or over-growth). The over-growth relates to the collagen in the skin, a protein that gives strength to its complex structure and prevents easy damage from rubbing, stretching, etc. Excess collagen becomes piled up as firm fibrous lumps – which can be much bigger than the original spots, varying from 1–2mm to 1cm or even bigger. The scars tend to last for years but in some cases will flatten off and shrink. Your skin type can also influence the chance of your getting this type of scarring – the darker your skin, the greater chance of your developing these scars.

Loss of skin tissue (sunken scars)

These are much more common than the raised scars, and show up as depressions or pits in the skin. There are several different types:

- **Ice-pick scars**. As the name suggests, these are like wounds from an ice-pick. They are small, with a jagged edge and steep sides, and usually occur on the cheeks.

- **Depressed scars**. These are larger ice-pick scars, with sharp edges and the same steep sides. The base of these larger scars is quite firm to the touch.

- **Soft scars** can be shallow or deep but are much softer. They tend to be small, and have much more gently sloping edges that merge into the normal skin.

- **Atrophic patches** are flat scars where the skin seems very shrunken and thin (atrophy). They are usually small on the face but can be 1cm or more on the body. The thin skin can look bluish at first but usually ends up as an ivory white colour with time.

- **Follicular macular atrophy** (small atrophic patches) is most likely to appear on the chest and back after extensive acne. It results from damage to the elastic fibres in the skin around the pores. These fibres normally keep the skin stretched and flat, so, where they are damaged, the skin bulges up into soft little lumps that often look like whiteheads. They can improve after months or years as the skin repairs the damage.

Before we look at the type of treatment available for scarring, remember a few facts about scars:

- You don't have to have severe acne to get scars.

- Squeezing at the 'wrong type' of spot (see the 'Which spots can I squeeze' guide at the end of Chapter 4, *Treatment from your GP*) will increase your chances of developing scars.

- Constant picking and poking at spots, especially with instruments such as metal nail files and tweezers, will increase your chances of developing scars.

- Scars may not appear until several years after your acne has gone; this is as a result of the skin losing its natural elasticity and starting to reveal the areas previously affected.

- Treating acne early will greatly reduce your chances of getting permanent, or at least very-hard-to-treat, scars.

Treating scars

There is mixed news here. If you are of the skin type most likely to scar as a result of acne, it may be that even the best physical treatment could leave you with different but just as ugly scars. You really have to spend a lot of time talking to people who have a special interest in acne and getting realistic answers about the relative benefits of the different types of treatment. Time and a little money spent at this phase will save you a fortune later. Talk to your GP, dermatologist and, if possible, a plastic surgeon who works at an NHS hospital. You might have to pay privately to consult a plastic surgeon but it will be a lot less than paying a private clinic to start treatment.

Treating the scars resulting from loss of tissue can involve anything that strips off layers of skin. This aims to bring all the skin down to the level of the lowest scar and then new skin growing without the scars. Various different techniques are used, ranging from chemicals to peel away layers (giving only a superficial effect), through sandpaper treatment which can go quite deep, to lasers which burn off layers of skin.

Getting a good result is difficult, especially for the pitted type of scarring. Sometimes only 35–50 per cent improvement is achieved, and you must ask yourself whether this would be enough to make you feel better, especially if coping with scars is very difficult for you. Treating scars should not just be the physical side of things – you will probably benefit from counselling before undergoing treatment, to appreciate the procedure and the realistic outcomes and how you will deal with the healing process and looking to the future. This can be done with a proper, in-depth consultation with the dermatologist or surgeon who will be undertaking the procedure and with the help of a trained counsellor or psychologist. How you deal emotionally with the procedure and the future may need further help from the counsellor or you might find 'self-improvement' books helpful in working through your feelings. Many people under-estimate the value of these books but, if you are prepared to make the time to read through and are sure that you want to 'move on', they can be very useful. A good bookstore, the internet or local library will have whole sections devoted to such books.

I'm from Jamaica and have keloid scars. What can I do about them?

The darker your skin, the more common keloids are, and they are difficult to treat. You probably have two options.

- An injection of steroid into the scar itself can help. It must be done by a doctor with experience of doing this, as it can cause a depressed pale scar if overdone. To try to prevent this side-effect, a series of small amounts is injected every two to three months.

- The other option is to try a silicon gel sheet. The sheet, which is thin, clear and flexible, sticks over the keloid and can be worn 12–14 hours a day. It is a little unclear how it works but there is some good scientific evidence of its success. This treatment can be prescribed by your doctor or you can buy it from your pharmacist/chemist shop.

I have developed brown blotches on my face where I used to have acne. Will they go away?

Yes, they will, but it could be months or years, depending on your skin type. The brown is extra pigment produced as a result of the inflammation in your skin and will gradually fade. There are some treatments that can help fade the marks but you should not try to treat them with any fading lotions you might see in the shops, as they could leave you with permanent lighter marks.

The treatments doctors prescribe for the blotches are often the same ones that can treat acne. Azelaic acid and the topical retinoids have a slow but good effect, and are often used together. Hydroquinone in a 5% solution is also used but it is more likely to affect your background skin colour, especially if it was dark to start with.

Even though my acne has cleared up after isotretinoin (Roaccutane) treatment, it still looks very red – almost sunburnt. Will this go?

Yes. The skin can look quite inflamed for weeks or months after Roaccutane treatment but settles back to normal. It goes red because of the acne inflammation itself and the irritant and drying effect of the drug. Keeping it well moisturised and using a soap substitute should help.

Vitamin E?

I have some deep scars left as a result of having acne on my temples. I have heard that vitamin E might help – what is your advice?

There is no evidence that vitamin E helps scars. However, most vitamin E creams are good moisturisers, and this can improve the quality of your skin in general and perhaps help make the scars less obvious.

Laser treatment

I went to a clinic to find out about laser treatment, but they said they couldn't promise me any results and that my skin might improve by only 30 per cent. This isn't much if I am forking out £3,000 – what do you suggest?

The jury is still out on lasers. A recent scientific review felt that there was insufficient evidence to recommend their use and some have side-effects of heating up the skin and causing inflammation. New 'cold' lasers may get round this problem but the figure of 30 per cent is quite realistic. Looking at it the other way round means that your scars will still be 70 per cent of what they were and it can be difficult to tell if you have achieved any benefit at all.

When I went to the laser clinic, I told them that I had recently finished a course of isotretinoin, and they said they can't help me until I have waited for a full 18 months. Why is this? Surely it has left my system by now?

This is frustrating, but good advice. The good work done by the isotretinoin carries on after you stop the treatment even though it has left your system completely by six weeks after a course ends. You also have quite young scars and this is an important point to consider when seeking any treatment for scarring. Scar tissue matures slowly and may take a good year, or sometimes longer, to reach its final state. Any treatment done while the scar tissue is still active and maturing could stimulate further scarring and make matters worse. A final thought is that you yourself may then be happier with your appearance and not want to pay a lot of money for relatively little benefit.

I am Asian and when I asked about laser treatment from the Acne Support Group they told me it wouldn't be suitable for my skin type as I might get pigment changes. What am I supposed to do?

Asian or African-Caribbean skin is very difficult to treat, because it is much more reactive than white skin – causing pigment changes after inflammation or damage. Laser treatment causes a lot of heat-related inflammation, which often results in large dark areas that you might find worse than the scars. There are some new 'cool' operating lasers that might be more suitable for your type of skin but we don't have very much experience with them yet.

I think it is terrible that I have to pay for laser treatment of my scars. To make it worse, the doctor told me that it was a 'cosmetic' problem. I'll give him 'cosmetic' – it almost destroyed my life! Why did he call it 'cosmetic' and why should I have to pay for it?

It is nothing to do with your GP or with the consultant who runs the laser clinic. Decisions like this are made at local or regional primary care organisation level. It is a sad fact that many ill-informed people in management positions can describe problems as cosmetic and decide not to fund them. If you can believe it, we may be better off in this country than in many places in Europe. France, for example, doesn't allow the prescription of any mois-turisers and some countries are even considering labelling all skin disease as 'cosmetic' so you wouldn't even get your acne treated by the health service. All people with skin problems should make sure that their MP knows of the misery caused, so that they will lobby to prevent any shrinkage of the service available on the NHS.

Creams

Ten years after I had terrible acne I am still suffering with scars and am trying a cream. Do you think it will help?

It is difficult to answer your question because we don't know what type of scars or skin colouring you have. Scars from extra tissue or from deep damage and loss of tissue will not be helped by creams. Some very superficial scars may look better if you keep your skin in good condition with a moisturiser, and can sometimes be improved by using the same retinoid creams that are prescribed to treat acne. They are stronger versions of 'anti-wrinkle' treatments and do seem to have some effect in encouraging the growth of new collagen to give strength to the skin.

If you do use a retinoid cream, you should avoid sunlight, so use a good suncream of at least 15 SPF, even on non-sunny days, to help protect your skin. You will usually have to use these creams or gels for a long time before you start to see any significant results, and then continue to use them.

Injections

I have seen an ad offering injections to treat sunken scars. Is it worth trying?

Sunken scars happen because of a loss of skin structure resulting from damage to collagen and other tissue 'building blocks'. The injections – of collagen or of artificial ingredients – are used to bulk up the skin under the scar and make it look flat. They can work quite well but are not permanent and need redoing every few months. Some of the artificial ingredients irritate the skin less than collagen and may last longer. If the scar is on part of the face where the facial muscles are used less (e.g. the forehead or temples), its benefits may last up to six or eight months. Another procedure involves taking some fat from another part of your body and injecting it under the scar. Once again, though, it is not permanent.

This treatment is not available on the NHS, so check out skin clinics to see if they have experience of treating acne scars using 'injectable dermal fillers'. Don't go to anyone who isn't thoroughly experienced, and expect to pay from £200.

Cryotherapy

My friend had some very cold spray treatment to her raised scars. What was this?

This was *cryotherapy* using a fine spray of liquid nitrogen. Nitrogen is a gas that is part of the air we breathe. It has a very low boiling point so is only liquid below −196°Celsius. It has to be kept in special reinforced and pressurised flasks to prevent it boiling away. Liquid nitrogen is used to treat several different skin problems. You may have heard people talking about having warts and verrucas frozen – it is the same stuff. It can be used to treat the raised scars, especially if they are quite new. It is only worth doing in people with white skin, as it kills off the

pigment-producing cells and tends to leave a pale area, which is
bad news for Asians and African-Caribbeans.

Surgery

Why can't I just have my scars cut out?

Most acne scars would not be improved by cutting them out,
because so much tissue would have to be removed that you
would need lots of stitches or even a skin graft. The exception is
if you have a few little ice-pick scars. These can be removed
using an instrument called a punch biopsy. It is basically like a
sharp scalpel blade that is rolled round into a cylinder and comes
in several different sizes. Small scars can be neatly removed,
leaving a circular hole. If this is then closed with one or two
stitches so that the line of the scar fits into a skin crease or runs
in the same direction as wrinkles might do, it will heal with an
almost invisible scar.

Some GPs may be experienced in this procedure but many will
not, so you might need to ask for a referral to a dermatologist or
plastic surgeon. This treatment might not be available on the
NHS in some parts of the country.

I don't want to have any more treatment for my scars – it hurts and doesn't really improve them. I'm still fed up but no one wants to help me.

The first half of your comment is very sensible, as it is an attitude
that could help a lot of people. There does come a time when you
have to accept that further treatment is just not worth it and
begin to come to terms with what your acne has left you. The second half shows how difficult that can be. Some years ago a
remarkable man called James Partridge set up a charity called
Changing Faces. He had been badly burned and, like you,
decided enough was enough and refused further plastic surgery.
He felt, quite rightly, that there must be thousands of people with
disfigurement, from whatever cause, who just wanted to get their

lives going again. Out of the charity came an NHS-funded service called Outlook, based in Bristol, to which any GP can refer patients. Trained counsellors and psychologists work with people using one-to-one and group sessions, and help them accept whatever has happened to them, work out whether their own reaction is normal or abnormal and help them move on.

If you can learn to accept the level of scarring you have and come to terms with it, you will find that other people also start to see the real you and anyone who stares at your scars is the one feeling awkward. Outlook's contact details are in the *Useful addresses* appendix.

Camouflage

Most of my scars are quite flat but still a different colour from my normal skin. What is the best way of covering them?

You need to consult a cosmetic camouflage service. Some hospital departments offer this but the biggest provision nationwide comes from the Red Cross. Specially trained make-up experts will look at your skin colour and design a mixture that matches it exactly. You are then taught how to apply it and 'fix' it so that it lasts all day. Your GP will have to refer you to the service. Once the right mixture has been found, you can get it all on prescription!

7
Emotional scars

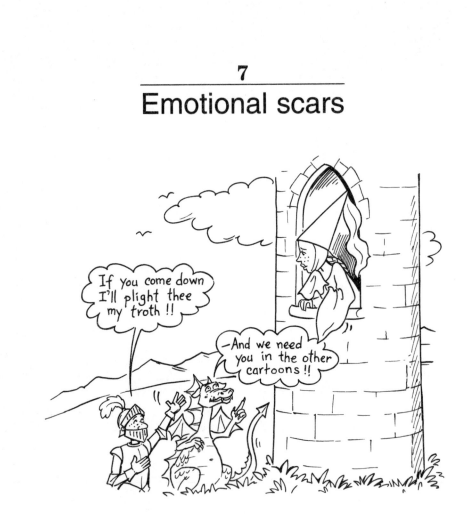

Introduction

'My daughter has literally shut herself in her room. She won't even come downstairs to join the family for dinner. Instead, I can hear her creep around after we have gone to bed. I am at my wits end with worry, but how can I speak to a closed door?'

If you have been reading through this book rather than dipping in and out, you should be getting a feeling that acne is not just a physical problem. It can have a profound effect on people that has no relation to the severity of the condition. The way you feel about yourself can mean that, if you are having a tough time anyway, even a few spots can cause problems.

It is only relatively recently that doctors, spurred on by patient support organisations such as the Acne Support Group, have started to look more seriously at the psychological effects of acne. There are many different ways in which these effects cause problems; some of the common ones are:

- social withdrawal,

- lowered self-esteem,

- reduced self-confidence,

- poor body image,

- embarrassment,

- feelings of depression,

- anger and aggression,

- preoccupation,

- frustration,

- higher rates of unemployment.

Of course, these effects are not felt on their own. One will often lead to another and another, and so on, each new problem feeding back into the first in a kind of downward spiral, leading to despair.

If you are lucky enough to get no more than a few spots, on the odd occasion, it is unlikely that you will feel the need to read this book. However, the Acne Support Group reports that many of its members may have only mild acne but are very deeply affected by it. Alternatively, your skin may have been under attack from acne for many years and shows the physical scars of your 'battle'. In other words, it doesn't matter whether you have the mildest or the most severe form of acne, it can affect you in a very deep and long-lasting way.

Reports of suicide as a direct result of acne are rarely reported, but suicidal feelings affect up to 15 per cent of Acne Support Group members. The very act of suicide may mean that someone hasn't been able to talk about their acne or problems associated with it. It could also be a hidden reason behind depression, often missed by a busy GP, who might only hear the words 'feeling down', 'not sleeping', 'not eating properly', 'feeling depressed' and not really look closer at the clues.

We all need to take responsibility for our own lives, but for some of us this is much harder than for others to achieve. Some people may resort to bottling up their feelings and literally lock themselves away, hiding their problems not only from the world but also from those closest to them, their family.

The majority of calls received at the Acne Support Group are from anxious mothers of teenagers who are bottling up their feelings and are defensive or rude in an attempt to deny they have a problem and to get well-meaning mothers off their backs. Sometimes it may seem better to deny you have a problem than say to yourself 'Right, that's it, I'm going to do something about this'. If you are a mother of such a teenager, you will know only too well what this may feel like. It's hard enough riding the emotional tidal waves of teenage years – they are the waves and you are often the little boat feeling helplessly tossed about. However, the advice that the Acne Support Group may give can be very helpful. If your teenager can't face talking about getting the acne treated but seems to show all the outward signs of being affected by it, why not write them a letter? This gives them a chance to read it in their own time, to digest, re-read and consider what you feel and how you want to help. A letter can also be torn up but, if that happens, you'll be no worse off than when you started. Anyway, that is what sticky tape was invented for!

The letter will also open a door (in some cases, literally) for them to discuss what they feel, if they want to. They may say nothing, but knowing that you have expressed your concerns and hopes for them will tell them that they are cared about and loved. It could make a small or a huge difference, but any difference could start a positive chain reaction. As long as the advice given is sound and based on facts given in this book, you are likely to have cracked what, at one stage, may have seemed like an impenetrable wall behind which your son or daughter stands feeling alone.

You and your acne

My doctor told me I needed to see a psychiatrist because I'm upset about my skin – he says the spots are not too bad. I say, get a life! I just want my skin cleared, not to have my head examined! Shall I just not go when the appointment comes?

One reason for your doctor suggesting that you visit a psychiatrist may be because of the way you are reacting to having acne. Most doctors are able to diagnose the type of acne you have (i.e. mild, moderate or severe) with little difficulty. It is possible that your doctor has graded your acne as mild but feels that you are reacting to it as if you have a more severe type. Perhaps he feels that you are showing signs of depression that could be helped by a psychiatrist. There is little to lose by keeping the appointment and spending a bit of time explaining your frustrations. Psychiatrists are not there to just examine your head, they are medical doctors who are qualified to help with conditions that may not be just physical. We hope that your doctor is also treating your skin – check through Chapter 4, *Treatment from your GP*, to see if you are on the best possible medication.

Whenever I look at magazines, they always have amazing-looking girls in them, with not a spot or blemish. If so many people have spots, how come they are not shown as well? I think it would give us some hope to think we are not the only people who get zits.

Oh, the power of the airbrush! If every model pictured were shown with a few spots, moles or lumps, magazines might not sell so well. So it is purely with sales, not reality, in mind that magazines want to portray their models as 'perfect'. Everyone will get a few spots or blackheads in their lives – there really are very, very few exceptions to this. Magazines are meant to inspire us, but in fact they, in their own way, lie to us too! Throw out the magazines until you feel your skin is improving. Look around you on the streets and you'll see that it is far more common to have spots than not.

My doctor told me I have dsymorphobia or something similar (can't quite remember) and told me to read up on it and stop wasting his time. Well, it's not my fault I have a face full of spots is it? I can't help picking them, they just have to go. I can't help being ugly but I wish I could just accept all this and get on with my life. If only the doctor would give me some treatment, I know I'd be all right. So why won't he give me any treatment?

It sounds as though you feel very frustrated and resentful, especially as you consider yourself to be 'ugly'. This is a classic sign of *dysmorphophobia*, which is the name for when someone is convinced they are ugly or deformed. It's quite similar to anorexia, when people look in the mirror and see someone very fat, when in fact they can be dangerously skinny. This condition is not easy to deal with and it may take some drug treatment and intensive counselling to help.

Treating the acne, even if it is mild, is very important to help you feel better about yourself but, from our experience, this will not always 'cure' the overall problem. It is possible that, if you remain dysmorphophobic, you will start to see other 'imperfections' on your face that seem big to you but won't to others. Don't give up on seeking help. Try contacting MIND (details in the *Useful addresses* appendix), and agreeing to seeing a psychologist or psychiatrist if your doctor suggests this.

If anyone looks at me, they stare at my spots. I am so ashamed and feel so dirty. I just cry all the time and I want to quit school because there's no point when all people do is stare. Where can I find a good doctor who will get rid of these spots once and for all? I am 17.

A 'good doctor' is any doctor who gives you the right help. Remember the good news that treating acne is much easier these days – your GP will know of lots of treatments that you can try. Take this book along with you if necessary and discuss your treatment options. Be sure to mention how having acne is making you *feel*. Giving up on school and dreams of a future career because of your acne now is not worth it.

It is easy to believe that we know what another person is thinking. Because you feel self-conscious, it is natural to assume that they are thinking badly of you but, if you were to stop and ask them what was going through their mind, you would often be surprised by their answer. Try making eye contact with people and holding their gaze; it can give you more confidence that they are looking at *you* and not your spots.

I can't face going into changing rooms in shops, especially when they don't have single rooms to get dressed in private. It really depresses me, as all I can see in the mirrors is my ugly, spotty skin staring at me. I even have acne on my back, so any clothes I buy have to cover all my back and shoulders. Are there any shops I can go to where I won't have to face this problem?

It's not possible to recommend certain shops, as they all vary in their changing room facilities. However, if you are feeling very self-conscious, you could try shopping by mail order so that you can try the clothes on in the privacy of your own home. In the meantime, get started on an acne treatment and stick to it for at least two months. When you start to see an improvement, you will find yourself regaining your confidence, and your fear of changing rooms will soon be a thing of the past.

I'm a 17-year-old boy and I just want to die because of my acne – it is all over my face and back. The doctors won't help and my mum keeps on bugging me to 'pull myself together'. No one knows what I am going through. Why can't anyone help?

Saying you want to die is a very big statement. Some people do want to die because of their acne and they feel so depressed and helpless. However, it may be worth looking at your mother's reaction as something that is aimed at helping, not bugging, you. Perhaps she is very concerned and feels quite helpless.

It is very understandable to feel you are the only one going through your experience. The Acne Support Group reports that up to 15 per cent of its members feel suicidal, but this is not to say they actually go ahead and take their life. There are a few things you can do to help yourself out of your 'negative spiral':

- Speak to someone today. Call the Samaritans, who are trained to help with people in your position. They will be able to give you undivided attention and a friendly listening ear. (Their number is in your local phone book.)

- Make the decision to get medical help for your skin *now* and to stick with the treatment. If the first treatment doesn't work, try another and another, until you get the right one. Be sure to tell your GP how your acne is affecting your life. The doctor needs to know how serious this is for you.

- Accept help from your mother, if you can. You may feel that she is 'bugging' you but ask her if this is really what she intends to do. You can be sure the answer to this is going to be 'no'. Talk to her about how she can help you.

My problem is that, according to all my friends and the doctor, I'm imagining I have spots. Well, I used to be a model and I had anorexia, but then I got hospitalised and, as I put on weight, I got some zits. Then for a year my zits got pretty bad – according to me, not anyone else. I have been to the doctor and she says they are over. According to my best friend my zits are only visible through a microscope, my brothers can't take me asking them every day . . . and my boyfriend says he doesn't notice anything. It's weird but I've let it control me totally, and I really can't take it. When I walk in the street, everybody looks at me and I feel so self-conscious; my mum says its 'cause I am pretty, but I keep thinking that if they see my zits they won't like me.

Some people sail through adolescence with nothing more than a few spots, and, if they get treatment, they may simply grow out of them. For others, it can be much harder to handle the changes of our bodies as we grow and develop, and I imagine you must be feeling very confused. No one ever truly knows what someone else is thinking, so when you say that if people see your zits they won't like you, you are only guessing. The truth is more likely to be that someone looking at you is thinking 'she's got nice eyes' or 'what shall I wear tomorrow night?'

You believe you have a problem with your spots even though everyone around you is telling you that you don't. Sometimes it is very tempting to keep asking, just to get someone to agree with you . . . which doesn't seem to be the case. The fact you have had anorexia gives us the feeling that you may still feel confused about your body and the mirror continues to 'lie'. If you don't get independent support, you could continue in this negative spiral and end up feeling quite depressed. There are many people who should be able to support you through this time, but family and close friends may not be the right ones just now. If you contact ChildLine or speak to someone at the Eating Disorders Association (details in the *Useful addresses* appendix), you will find a sympathetic ear. We also suggest that you return to your doctor to explain how badly you feel. Perhaps you could ask her to refer you to a counsellor, who could also help.

I get pimples and I just *have* to squeeze them. I squeeze them with tweezers, which I can't throw away because I have to pluck my eyebrows. I hate doing it but I just do and I look so ugly, so can you please tell me what to do?

You probably already know the answer to this problem: the tweezers must go! It is very tempting to pick and poke at your skin to try to get rid of a blemish or spot, but you are very likely to damage the skin permanently because you are not letting it settle or expel the spot naturally. The good news is that there are *some* spots you can gently squeeze (see the 'Traffic light guide to squeezing spots' at the end of Chapter 4), but the skin is delicate and should be treated with respect. If you still want to pluck your eyebrows but don't trust yourself with the tweezers, ask your mum to look after them and get into the habit of giving them straight back once you've used them.

I am really getting fed up with my spots. I am 16 and I used to feel quite attractive and had a few boyfriends. But in the last year my skin seems to have got worse than ever and I haven't had a boyfriend for ages. Sometimes I just stay at home even when my friends go out, because I feel so ugly and ashamed. My mum says it is because I eat too many chocolate bars, but I don't really. She says I should wash more often (I wash at least three times every day) but my friend at school said I should go to the chemist to get some creams. I don't want to be like this forever. Why me?

What a lot of advice you've been given! You must be feeling quite confused about why you have spots. Chapter 2, which deals with the causes of acne, should be very helpful, not just for you but also for the people who have been giving you well-meaning – but incorrect – advice. Lots of people ask 'why me?' for every disease that exists, but it is nothing you have done that has caused your acne.

The most positive step you can take now is to go to your GP and seek treatment. Once your skin starts to improve, it is inevitable that your confidence will return. Meeting boys and going out with friends is all about confidence, and if you feel you are starting to get more control over your skin, you will begin to feel better about yourself. You won't be like this forever.

I have had acne since I was 14. I am now 26 and feel thoroughly fed up. Why do I have to put up with the constant misery of spots and the scars they are now starting to leave? My doctor is little help – she has tried some antibiotics but has now told me that, if they haven't worked, nothing will. Can this be true?

How disappointed you must feel! To be told that there is no further help is simply not true. Your doctor may feel that she has exhausted the list of possible treatments, but in fact she can prescribe a combination of over 100 treatments, so I am sure the options have all not been fully explored.

You have had acne for 12 years, which is a very long time, and you are starting to see scarring. We think it is time for you to talk about visiting a dermatologist, continuing to use a treatment from your doctor while you wait for the appointment. Don't despair: stick to your guns, learn all you can about your skin and the treatments, and make sure that you see the people who can help.

My doctor has suggested that I see a psychologist. What use will that be? I want my skin to be better, not to talk about it?

Psychologists don't just talk to you. They help you look at your reaction to a situation to try to see whether it is a normal or an abnormal one. If feeling the way you do about your acne is normal, they can help you deal with this and get on with the your life without allowing your skin problem to get in the way. If it is an abnormal reaction, they will work with you to try to change it so that you can cope better with your skin.

A lot of psychology deals with accepting a problem, coming to terms with it and getting on with your life. It is very normal to feel upset and cross that you have acne, and a psychologist will not try to change this but, rather, will help you to accept it.

Make sure that you are also getting the best skin treatment available, as this will probably work better if you don't feel so stressed out.

I am writing to you with tears in my eyes. I really can't stand my damn face any more – it is so ugly and my spots are really so disgusting I sometimes just want to die. I've got rid of all my mirrors because I was always looking in them and picking at my skin.

Spots, acne, zits – whatever you want to call them, they can all seem very ugly. Mirrors can seem like your worst enemy if you are affected by acne but, if you get help for your skin, you should find that within the next six weeks you will be ready to put the mirrors back up, as you watch your skin improve. Remember: if the first treatment doesn't work, keep trying until you find one that does. Having acne is not a reason to want to die, especially when it is so treatable. While you are waiting for your treatment to work, why not talk to someone you feel you can trust. You'll be amazed how it can help to share feelings that have been bottled up.

The family

Please can you help? My son has taken to going out only at night-time, like some sort of vampire. He hates bright lights and hangs his head low, hidden behind quite long, messy hair. His acne is really quite bad, but every time I ask him what he is going to do about it, he just grunts or, worse, shouts at me to mind my own business. He is 16.

You can almost sum up the main reason for his behaviour in the last sentence. He is 16, and this is a hard enough age to cope with, let alone being burdened by acne. The long hair you describe and avoiding eye contact indicate that he wants to hide away – an attitude adopted by many teenagers not wishing to stare the world boldly in the eye. The bright lights help focus attention on the skin, so avoiding daylight will all be part of his 'coping' strategy.

Being told to mind your own business when you are merely concerned can be very hurtful and no doubt he wants to give you the message that you are not needed. Trying to deal with this sort of behaviour is challenging but it is worth sticking at your attempts to help. Perhaps, though, you can change the way you do it. As suggested in the introduction to this chapter, consider writing to your son and letting him see that you want to help. Leaving some acne leaflets, like those the Acne Support Group produce, within easy reach might give him a chance to read them. It is, however, impossible to force someone to do something against their will. So, no matter how much you may want to help right now, it may simply be a matter of sitting it out until he either helps himself or comes to you for advice.

My daughter is a really beautiful, attractive girl. She was so full of life until about six months ago, when she started to become obsessed with her skin. She does get some spots (don't all teenagers?), but she doesn't seem able to cope with them at all. When she comes home from college, she literally runs upstairs and spends half an hour looking in the mirror, picking at her face. I feel so helpless. Please reassure me that this is just a phase.

It probably is just a phase – but a difficult one for all the family, as it is likely that your daughter's behaviour is affecting you all. Some people seem to take a few spots in their stride and accept it as part of normal teenage life, whereas others may simply become paranoid or withdrawn. The picking is a sign that she is particularly anxious, and this may become an obsession if the mirror and picking sessions become more prolonged. If you feel she could be becoming 'obsessed', the organisation Obsessive Action may be able to help (contact details in the *Useful addresses* appendix).

My daughter is about to sit her A levels. She has been studying very hard for them but she has taken to locking herself in her room, full of misery over a few spots. This is such a vital time for her – exam results mean everything these days – I am at my wits' end. I have tried to tell her that it is nothing and her exam results are important, but she won't listen. I need advice.

The stress of studying and worrying about her exams has made her acne flare up. Anything you can do to help her relax is likely to help her spots – perhaps avoid mentioning the importance of the exams for the time being. She will also want to carry on having a life despite the studying and must be finding it harder to cope with the flare-up at this time. She seems to be being deprived of the chance to socialise and relax, returning refreshed to her studies. Try to let her know that you understand this, and encourage her to see her doctor, who may well be able to prescribe her suitable treatment, or alter her current treatment and thus improve things for her.

My brother is really starting to be affected by his acne, which is really bad. He has stopped going out with his friends and he stays in his room for ages. Every time Mum tries to talk to him, he just shouts at her and tells her to mind her own business. Can you tell me why he is so bothered about his skin, when, to me and Mum, it doesn't seem that bad?

The way we see ourselves is often very different from how others see us. From the way your brother is shouting at your mum, it sounds as though he is very frustrated, and her concern may be coming across to him as 'interfering'. In truth, many teenage boys find it hard to talk about their spots. It is a very embarrassing subject for them and often they would prefer not to be reminded about it, even if the advice is well meaning. It might help if you or your mum were to write him a letter that he can read in his own time, explaining how concerned you are and give him a copy of this book or the information pack from the Acne Support Group.

He can then make his own choices and, with luck, he will see that you are acting from kindness and concern.

My brother has terrible acne but, to be honest, he doesn't seem to care about it. He is starting to get some scars and he doesn't go out much. What can I do to help?

The fact you describe him as not going out much suggests that perhaps he is more bothered than he is letting on. Some people don't seem to be bothered by acne, even when in some cases it is quite severe. We suspect, though, that this is more of a way of coping with acne – literally putting on a brave face. In other cases, it may be that the person has great inner confidence and is not upset or affected by their outer appearance. Good for them! But for those who are upset and choose not to show it, it can be quite emotionally unhealthy for them. Bottling up emotions and not treating acne are ingredients for potentially longer-term emotional problems. If you would like to help your brother, why not leave this book lying around the house where he can easily pick it up? Even starting off a conversation with 'I care about you enough to tell you . . .' might be worth a try.

Friends

My friend used to be so easy going, but a couple of girls in our class have been teasing her and calling her 'Braille head' because of the spots she has across her forehead. Now my friend is growing her fringe and is starting to get really upset. Can you help?

It's hard to hide away from having acne, but growing a fringe over the spot-affected area is not going to help – in fact, if she uses hair oils or wax, it may make it worse! Your friend is lucky to have someone who cares about her, and it is worth reminding her that you are there to support her. Unfortunately, too many people are called names, often for the most minor 'abnormalities' but, if the teasing continues, it might be worth speaking to a teacher you trust. This sort of teasing can also lead to bullying, but there are some great websites that include tips on dealing with this sort of behaviour. A couple are listed at the end of Appendix 1, *Useful addresses*.

My best mate just keeps on about her spots all the time, which is really boring and gets on my nerves. She doesn't even have that many spots – like only one or two – but she always picks them, and goes to the mirror every break to check out her face. I told her last week that she is obsessed, but she said I didn't know what it was like and to get lost. She hasn't spoken to me since. Should I just ignore her?

It can be hard to put up with a friend's behaviour that makes little sense to you. However, she seems to be acting as if her few spots are a real bother to her. Take her aside and tell her that, as her friend, you are a little bored with hearing her complaints when, in fact, there are loads of treatments she can get from her doctor. She probably needs reassurance from you, which is why she is constantly going on about her skin, so try to be patient and supportive. She will feel much better once her skin is cleared.

At school or work

It's hard to believe, but the bully of our class, a real loud mouth called Ben, has the worst case of zits you've ever seen! I think it's amazing that he has the cheek to tease others about being fat or smelly when he has the most disgusting spots himself!

This is a classic case of bully or be bullied. It is possible that he is self-conscious of his acne, and has chosen to turn this situation around to bully others – to almost dare them to tease him. Bullying is a sign of weakness, even though it may be very scary to be on the receiving end of it. Ben needs to get help for his acne if he doesn't want it to scar (especially if it is a bad case), but he is probably going to be very resistant to friendly approaches. It is going to be down to him to realise he needs to get his skin treated but perhaps you can help subtly by leaving the website address of the Acne Support Group (see the *Useful addresses* appendix) lying around.

When I got my apprenticeship at the factory, I was really pleased. But when I was called 'pizza face' on my first day at work I was really not happy. On the outside, I just laughed it off, but four months later they are still calling me 'Pizza' and not my real name. Who should I complain to about this, or am I going to lose my job if I do? Maybe I should just not get bothered about it all.

In response to a survey run by the Acne Support Group in 1997, about 27 per cent of its members said they were still teased in the workplace because of having acne. This sort of teasing is often taken for granted, especially in an all-male environment, when it's just a 'lads thing'. This doesn't mean you have to stand for it, though. Report your concerns to your manager or personnel/ human resources, saying that you would like to work together to resolve the situation. And when you are next called 'Pizza', don't react at all. Tell your colleagues your name and say that is what you would like to be called. They are likely to lose interest if you show no reaction to being called 'Pizza'.

Remember to get your acne treated, and watch them wonder why they ever called you this ridiculous and childish name!

8
Complementary and alternative treatment

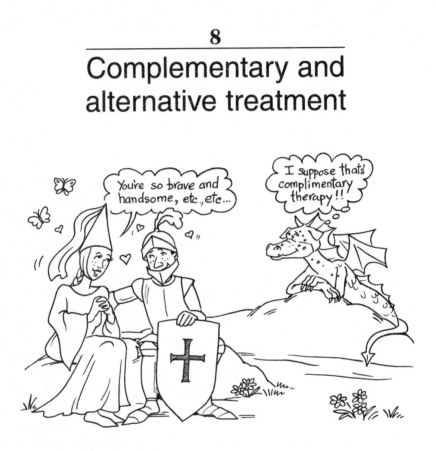

Introduction

'I like the fact that when I visited the homoeopath he really seemed to sit and listen and spent ages taking down my life story. I felt I had, at last, spent time with someone who cared'.

It's true that many people seek medical help from someone other than their GP, spending money in the hope of finding relief from symptoms that have made their life miserable. Acne is no exception to this, especially as it may take time and patience to see results from treatment.

Some 25 per cent of people with acne try complementary medicines. 'Complementary medicine' is a good term because it reflects the way that the treatment or therapy can sit alongside more traditional treatment rather than replacing it altogether. 'Alternative treatments' are just that, suggesting a more radical change of treatment without a sense of partnership between you, your GP and another practitioner. We much prefer the complementary approach, as it can be a great help to you while you continue with your prescribed treatment.

Much of the problem with different approaches to treatment comes from the lack of scientific study that provides evidence of the value of the standard creams and tablets, but this doesn't always matter. Treatments such as reflexology and aromatherapy may have no scientific evidence of success in treating acne but they are very good at making you feel better and more relaxed. Stress is a major cause of a flare-up of acne for some people, and any treatment that helps you relax could be worth trying.

A whole range of different approaches to helping you cope with acne are available outside the NHS, and many practitioners are genuinely trying to improve the quality of life of their clients. Sadly, though, there are people and clinics that make exaggerated claims for their particular approach or product. There is little government regulation of this, although a recent report from the Associate Parliamentary Group on Skin has looked at what can be done to help protect consumers by using existing Trading Standards legislation or by giving the Medicines Control Agency a wider brief. The latter proposal would mean that all complementary and alternative treatments on offer would have to be registered with this official government organisation, whose strict regulations are already well known among ethical pharmaceutical companies!

Many products that are advertised in magazines, newspapers and the internet could have real promise but they are not subject to proper controls or evaluation, so it is very difficult to judge which ones are worth trying. Anyone who has got better after using a different treatment will be very positive about it but it is human nature not to say when a treatment has failed, especially if you paid a lot of money for it!

It is also worth noting that many companies, especially those offering 'treatments' on the internet, do not examine your skin or, in some cases, take a medical history. Such questions help medical doctors decide what treatment may be best for you, and there is a risk that important information could be missed in the rush to find a 'cure'.

The Cochrane Group is an organisation set up to study the evidence for many treatments used in the NHS, and will soon be reporting on complementary treatments for acne. It will be worth keeping an eye on their website (details in the *Useful addresses* appendix). We are sure that proper studies will reveal that some treatments are as good as conventional ones and might be better tolerated. But GPs and dermatologists need to be certain of the science behind a treatment before they advise people to use it, as they are much more easily held to account if things go wrong.

Safety

As well as looking for evidence of benefit, we also need to look at the safety of complementary or alternative treatment. It may not really matter if you choose to spend money on a useless safe treatment. However, if a treatment does you harm, the NHS has to pick up the bill to repair the damage. Every year brings new reports of people dying or being made ill by herbal remedies – both Chinese and Western – so you must think carefully before choosing your complementary or alternative practitioner.

Most complementary practitioners work privately and are better than NHS doctors at 'selling' their treatment. It is essential, therefore, to be very careful when choosing whom to see and what advice and treatment to trust. Speaking to someone who calls him- or herself a 'consultant' may mean nothing as far a professional qualification is concerned; add a white coat and an air of authority and you may find yourself lulled into a false sense of security. Professional bodies regulate many of the forms of complementary therapy and qualifications can be checked, so ask the practitioner for details of his or her training and accreditation. If they have studied hard and achieved certificates to prove their training, they should be very proud to show them to you.

The Royal College of Nursing has produced some guidelines to help you to choose a reliable practitioner. They are given below.

Ask the following questions:

- What are his/her qualifications and how long was the training?

- Is he/she a member of a recognised, registered body with a code of practice?

- Can he/she give you the address and telephone number of this body so that you can check?

- Is the therapy available on the NHS?

- Can your GP delegate care to the practitioner?

- Will he/she keep your GP informed in the same way that a hospital consultant would?

- Is this the most suitable complementary medicine for your condition?

- Are the records confidential?

- What is the cost of treatment?

- How many treatments will be needed?

Then ask yourself:

- Did the practitioner answer your questions clearly and to your satisfaction?

- Did the practitioner give you information to look through at your leisure?

- Did the practitioner conduct him/herself in a professional manner?

- Did the practitioner make excessive claims about the treatment?

The Acne Support Group has advised its members also to consider the following suggestions:

- If you feel under pressure to commit yourself at the initial consultation, you should be suspicious. Just like deciding to purchase a car, you should be allowed time to think and consider your options. If necessary, you should be able to go home and take your own time to decide without feeling the pressure to leave a deposit (which may be hard to get back if you decide not to go ahead).

- Take a friend with you and ask their honest opinion of the whole experience, the clinic, the person you spoke to, the claims they made etc. Sometimes it is easy to feel so desperate that you will believe anyone. Your friend will have your best interests at heart; the clinic or practitioner will have their own best interests at heart (although this doesn't mean they aren't professional)!

- Is the clinic or practitioner willing to let you speak to people they have helped with acne? Speaking to someone about their experience may help you make your decision; you can ask the nitty gritty questions like 'Did it hurt?' and 'Did it really work?'

- If you feel you are being blinded by science, ask them to stop and explain in plain English. If someone gave you instructions to get from A to B and you didn't understand them, you would ask – so make sure you do the same here, especially as it is your face that is in their hands!

It is best to avoid any practitioner who:

- claims to cure skin diseases,

- advises you to stop conventional treatment without consulting your GP,

• makes you feel uncomfortable – you need a good relationship to ensure full benefit from any treatment.

Aromatherapy

My friend tells me that she really loves having an aromatherapy massage, and has suggested that I go with her next time. Is it safe for me to have an aromatherapy massage with acne?

Yes, it can be if you discuss it carefully with the aromatherapist. You shouldn't have any massage on areas where you have acne or have recently had it, as it could clog the pores up even more, unless the aromatherapist has oils suitable for skin with acne such as tea tree or lavender. Make sure that the oil used is a light one . . . and enjoy it. As with other techniques that involve touch, this in itself can be very enjoyable, especially if you find that other people tend to recoil from touching you when they see your acne.

Reflexology

A cousin keeps raving about reflexology. What is it, and can it help?

Reflexology is a massage therapy that uses acupuncture points on the feet that represent different parts of the body. The feet are massaged using talcum powder and you don't need to take any other clothes off if you are self-conscious about your skin. The contact can in itself be beneficial and it is another good way to relax and feel more able to cope with having acne. This actually seems able to influence the condition, as a positive attitude can help your body fight it.

Hypnotherapy

A friend 'cured' her smoking with hypnotherapy. Would it work at all with my acne?

Hypnotherapy may help by relaxing you and giving you a more positive approach to the condition, thus making it easier for you to cope with your acne. It can work well if you are a picker and squeezer, because suggestion under hypnosis will help you to break this habit. However, hypnotherapy is not a treatment for acne, so you should still continue with treatment (or seek treatment) from your GP.

Homoeopathy

One of my friends says that I should try homoeopathy but I don't know what it is. Would it help my acne?

Homoeopathy is an approach to medicine in which it is believed that the symptoms of a disease are caused by the body's way of fighting the disease. Homoeopaths try to alter this effect by stimulating the healing mechanisms using special remedies. The remedies are based on substances that might produce the same symptoms (e.g. spots and inflammation) but are diluted many, many times so that no more than a trace of the substance is left. The treatment is safe and usually free from side-effects, although it can sometimes produce a flare-up if the wrong dilution is used first. Acne is a condition that can be helped by homoeopathy if used by experienced practitioners.

Remember to give the treatments you are prescribed at least two months to work. If, however, after this period of time, you do not see a noticeable improvement, you should ask for a different treatment or accept that homoeopathy may not be suitable for you on this occasion.

My local chemist sells homoeopathic remedies. Can I just ask his advice and buy one?

No, this is not the way to start homoeopathic treatment. A homoeopath will look at you as a person and decide what type of constitution you have. This takes into account how you react to things and what type of personality you have, helping to decide which remedy you should be given.

I'd quite like to see a homoeopath for my acne. Is it very expensive?

As with any alternative or complementary medicine, there are no fixed charges, so, if you see someone privately, you need to establish the total cost up front.

It might cost you nothing to see a homoeopath, as it is one branch of complementary medicine that is available in the NHS. There are five homoeopathic hospitals in the UK – Bristol, Glasgow, Liverpool, London and Tunbridge Wells. These hospitals are often staffed by local GPs who have a special interest and qualifications, but you will need to be referred by your own GP as you would be to any other NHS hospital. If you feel it is too far for you to travel to one of these hospitals, contact the Society of Homoeopaths or the British Homoeopathic Association (listed in the *Useful addresses* appendix) for details of local practitioners. One of the advantages of NHS homoeopathic hospitals is that the doctors working there have to look at how successful the treatment is and publish regular audits. It seems that homoeopathy works well for about half the people who try it.

If I decide to try homoeopathic remedies, how long would I have to take them?

Homoeopaths like to see you for an initial consultation and then for three or four follow-up appointments. This should take a total of about six months. As with other acne treatments, there is a lag time of around two months before they begin to show results but, if you respond, the six months of treatment should be enough.

Do the homoeopathic hospitals offer any other complementary treatment on the NHS?

You would have to ask them, as it varies both for what is on offer and for what your local primary care organisation will pay for. The Royal London Homoeopathic Hospital, for example, offers nutritional medicine, acupuncture and autogenic training (see the next question and answer) in addition to homoeopathy.

Autogenic training

I heard someone talking about autogenic training for their acne. What is it, and could it help me?

This is, perhaps, the one therapy that takes the effects of stress most seriously and tries to help you deal with it. When you are very stressed, you release hormones such as adrenaline, which speeds up your heart rate, and cortisol, a natural steroid that prepares your body to withstand injury. Remember that stress for our ancestors was a response to real physical danger, so the hormones released prepared them for 'fight or flight' – to stay and fight the danger or to run away. These hormones can cause you to produce more sebum, which is why they can make acne worse. Autogenic training teaches you a series of mental exercises and meditations that help you to 'switch off' the stress hormones. This can take eight weekly sessions of about an hour and continued home practice until your stress levels are back to normal and stay there.

This form of treatment is not widely available.

Other approaches

I went to a Harley Street practice where I saw this man who told me I have to take some herbs in a foul-smelling drink. It is very expensive and he won't tell me how long I'll need to take it. Do you think it will work?

No, is the quick answer. You have a right to know what is in any treatment you are given and what you should expect from it. The only thing we are certain about is that you will end up wasting a lot of money.

I tried cod liver oil to help my acne but, instead, I found that my skin seemed to get more oily. I was taking quite a high dose. Does cod liver oil affect the production of sebum or should I just take a lower dose?

There is no evidence that cod liver oil affects the production of sebum, although some members of the Acne Support Group have reported that, like you, they find their skin tends to become more greasy.

It could be thought to be worth a try because of its content of vitamin A but there is no evidence of any benefit in acne. It's worth remembering the two-month rule: if you see an improvement within this period of time, fine, but if you think your acne is getting worse or there is no noticeable improvement, you can consider this supplement to be of little or no benefit. Bin it, and move on. It should be quite safe to take alongside conventional acne treatments, so it is best to consider this as a complementary treatment.

I used neat tea tree oil on my face because I had read that it was safe to do so. However, my skin really burnt and turned red in the area I had applied it, and really dried out. Why did it do this?

We hope your skin has recovered. This is one of the few essential oils that can be used directly on the skin but, like other creams and lotions, it must always be used sparingly and, if necessary, you should build up tolerance by using it only once a day. Tea tree oil can be used neat on the skin but some people find that it is hard to tolerate and can cause the redness you describe. You can help relieve this by applying plenty of oil-free moisturiser to the area. Keep applying it until the skin has 'mopped up' as much as it can (this may mean applying it five or six times in a day). With this reaction in mind, it would be sensible to avoid using tea tree oil neat on your face in the future.

Where did you read that it was safe? This is a good example of the bad advice that you can find if you don't question the credentials of whoever is giving it or you haven't enough information. It also shows that 'natural' products can be very irritant and toxic, and should never be assumed to be safe. Some of the most poisonous substances on Earth are 'natural'! The face is a very sensitive part of the body, so anything that is new to you should be tried on a very limited area to start with in case you have another reaction.

There is evidence that tea tree oil can be useful in acne and compares well with benzoyl peroxide in some studies. However, the only study that had enough patients in it to be significant used a 5% strength, which wasn't as good as 5% benzoyl peroxide. Slightly stronger concentrations may well be worth using but they would be no better than the treatments already available from your GP.

I was given Zineryt for my acne. It contains zinc and I saw some zinc supplements in the health food shop. Would it be OK to take these?

This is a good question. As discussed in Chapter 4 (*Treatment from your GP*), Zineryt does contain zinc and the manufacturers have evidence that it helps prevent resistance, improves skin healing and keeps the antibiotic in contact with the skin for longer. This is when it is applied to the skin rather than taken by mouth, so tablets wouldn't necessarily have the same effects.

The zinc story may be more involved than this, as studies have found that zinc levels can be low in people with acne, and rise after treatment whether or not it included zinc. One such study used Zineryt (which also contains erythromycin) on its own and in combination with other treatments. There were only 26 patients in this study but it did find that zinc levels rose after treatment, the biggest rise being achieved with Zineryt plus an antibiotic. Other small studies have also found that taking zinc supplements can help. Larger scale studies are needed to see how effective zinc really is. But a small zinc supplement is safe to take and might help.

Why zinc is low and rises after treatment is not known, so we still have more to learn about acne.

I have heard that soybeans can help acne. Should I eat more of this food?

We haven't come across any evidence that eating soybeans (or soya beans) can help acne. What you might have heard about is the report of a very small study, suggesting that a moisturiser containing soya can help acne: it reduced the number of inflamed spots and general redness, and was thought to be starting to reduce the numbers of comedones. The study lasted only 35 days, so the researchers could not be sure of its long-term effects; a bigger and longer-lasting study is needed to look at this further. Soya contains what are called phyto-oestrogens. These are plant versions of the female hormone oestrogens, so the moisturiser might work by altering the effect of androgens on the skin and thus reducing the production of sebum.

Everyone tells me I have acne because of what I eat. I don't think I eat too many greasy things – should I see a nutritionist for treatment?

We cannot say often enough that diet has *no connection* with acne. You may well hear people saying they have changed what they eat and their acne has got better. Medical literature is full of anecdotes like that, and there are bound to be people who have an individual reaction to certain foods – we are all different. Health food shops, nutritionists and herbalists will promote foods and supplements that are supposed to treat acne but you will generally be wasting your money.

One thing that *is* worth doing about your diet is to make sure it is well balanced while allowing yourself treats. Having acne is bad enough without making life miserable by avoiding the foods you like! Include good sources of zinc (wholemeal bread, meat), vitamin A (carrots, liver) and polyunsaturated fats (spreading margarine, cooking oils). This will ensure that your general health is as good as possible and that your body is well able to repair the damage that acne can cause. This is particularly important if you are on a long course of antibiotics. Fruit and vegetables contain the anti-oxidant vitamins C and E, and these will help you fight infections.

9

Sex, growing up and practical concerns

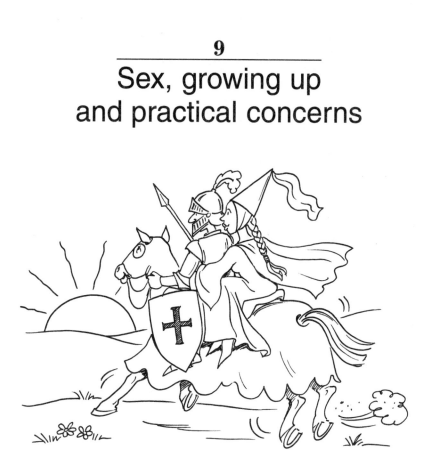

Introduction

'Having to give up on my dream of being an air hostess just because of my acne has devastated me.'

When you are 10 years old the world usually seems to be a safe place. Family and friends are supportive and provide you with shelter, food and love – the basics for us all. However, get to 15 years old and this picture may seem very different. As part of moving towards independence it is normal to start pushing at boundaries and trying to create a sense of 'self'. We question the rules of living at home, eat too much or too little, and turn our noses up at balanced meals, favouring instead fast food and quick calorie hits such as chocolate. Adults become people to be distrusted, and a sense of 'knowing it all' gets in the way of our seeking or accepting advice. The question of love still needs answers: do they, don't they, do I, don't I? Before you know it, life seems quite complicated. Throw acne on top of it all and you start to see why the teenage years can be so difficult.

It's also the time you start to think about the opposite sex – and having sexual relationships. It's merely cruel coincidence that this sex drive starts to kick in just as spots start to crop up. Many people mistake thoughts of sex or sexual activity as the cause of acne, but, as mentioned in Chapter 2 (**What causes acne?**), it is clear that the two are not linked. This doesn't stop some people feeling unattractive or self-conscious and affecting the way they feel about their bodies.

Parents think it is their right to give advice on all aspects of life, from fashion – 'You're not going out dressed like that?' – to hygiene – 'Have you washed your face this week?' but often their well-intentioned advice is seen as nothing more than interference and thus smelly Tom earns his reputation or fat Sally feels victimised. It's the same with getting acne. Parents' advice may not always be 100 per cent accurate, but it is well meaning and designed to help sort out the problem.

This chapter looks at these problems as well as others that occur as you grow older and still have acne.

Hormones, sex and pregnancy

I haven't started my periods yet but I've got loads of zits across my forehead and cheeks. Does this mean my periods will start soon? Will they go when my period comes?

Puberty doesn't always have a strict running order. Body hair, periods, acne, and growing and changing shape happen at different stages. It is possible that acne is the first sign for you, whilst for someone else it could be sweating or developing breasts. No one is able to predict when you will start your periods but acne is still one of the obvious signs of your body changing. Speak to your parents or a friend you trust about any worries, and you will probably realise that it is all a matter of patience. The forehead and cheeks are often the first place affected by spots. Use this book to guide you through treatments for them and let nature run its course.

I've heard that, if you have sex, it will make your skin start to get really spotty. Is that really true?

No, it's not true – it's just one of the myths that abound. The idea might have begun because we think about, or start to have, sexual relationships around the time of late puberty – the classic time for acne to start kicking in. But it's just one of nature's coincidences that they happen at roughly the same time.

I am 15 and I have started to think about sex quite a lot but I notice that I am getting a lot of spots, too. Are the two connected?

The two things are connected only by their common cause. Your body is maturing normally, so you are producing more adult levels of sex hormones. It is normal to think more about sex and, as almost all teenagers will get some degree of acne, that too is normal. Thinking about sex will make no difference to your acne, and, what is more, treating your acne will have no effect on your sexual development.

I've still got acne but also have a boyfriend who loves me and we want to start having sex. Can I go on the pill?

This is a difficult one to answer, as it depends on your acne and the type of treatment you are on. It is also worth saying that family planning experts recommend using condoms as a protective barrier against infection as well as contraception. Chapter 2, *What causes acne?*, deals with hormones and the pill – it may be that you can help your acne and have contraception as well with the form of pill called Dianette. Antibiotics can sometimes interfere with the way the pill works, so, if you are taking any, make sure your doctor or family planning clinic knows this. They will also help you choose a pill that will not make your acne worse.

My partner and I are planning on starting a family. Do I have to stop all my acne treatment if I get pregnant?

The biggest danger to the baby is from retinoids, either topically or by mouth. This includes adapalene, which is a retinoid-like drug. You should stop using these before you even start trying to get pregnant, as they affect the way a baby develops in the womb. The other topical treatment to avoid is azelaic acid, but the rest are thought to be safe. If you need to take antibiotics by mouth, erythromycin is safe but even this is better avoided in the first three months of pregnancy.

You must talk to your doctor about this in case there are particular problems relating to your health.

Work prospects

How long will I have acne? I want to join the army, which I have had my heart set on since as long as I can remember, but I don't want to be the only one with zits and get bullied for it.

Unfortunately, no one can tell you exactly how long you will have acne. If you have set your heart on joining the army, you need to let your doctor know and make sure you are on the best possible treatment. In Chapter 2 we mentioned the problems of friction from rucksacks and humidity, as these can make acne much worse. Until recently, the army used to refuse anyone with acne, or a history of bad acne, but pressure from the Acne Support Group and other patients' organisations has made them change this policy.

When I went for an interview to be an air stewardess, they told me I had good qualifications for the job, and I really thought I would get in. But my acne was really bad that day (probably not helped by stress of the interview) and I am convinced I didn't get asked back for a second interview because of it. First, can I get them to tell me if that is the case, and, second, can I sue them if this is the reason I didn't get offered the job?

It is impossible to know why you weren't offered the job. Some companies have very strict policies about who they recruit but it will seldom be based on acne. However, there are exceptions to this rule, especially if appearance is an important part of the job. It's a sad fact of life that this happens and you would have to be able to prove that you were treated unfairly to pursue it on a legal basis.

It is possible that you were turned down for perfectly legitimate reasons, such as there were so many good candidates, all with suitable qualifications, that the company might have had to be really tough with their choice. They may have noticed your stress and therefore felt that you might not be the most suitable candidate to handle what can be a very stressful job. Try to be positive and accept this decision. Get your acne treated, and don't give up on pursuing the career you want just because you didn't get through this time. Once your acne is cleared, you may wish to re-apply and then see if you are accepted.

I'm a trainee chef and work in a kitchen where it's really hot and humid. Is there anything I can do to help stop my pores getting blocked up?

This is difficult because the nature of the work means that you are bound to feel the effects of your working environment on your skin, and preventing your pores getting blocked will be very hard. The humidity produced from steaming food will probably make any pre-existing acne worse. So the following tips might be helpful:

- As often as possible, work near an open window, or ask for a window to be opened when it becomes very hot and humid.

- Take a cleanser with you to work and, on toilet breaks, use this to refresh your skin and to remove surface grease and sweat. Alternatively, you could wash your face with a mild soap.

- It is advisable to avoid wearing foundation or powder that might help block the skin pores. Try to leave them as clear as possible while you are working.

My son wants to be a motor mechanic. Won't all that grease make his acne worse?

First, you don't mention whether your son is taking any medication for his acne, which would be the first thing we would advise. Secondly, there is a type of acne called *mechanical acne*, which can be caused by working with industrial oils and greases that come into contact with the skin. Therefore it is very important to ensure that your son avoids as much unnecessary contact with any motor oils as he can. He should take his usual cleanser or mild soap to work to use to remove any oils as soon as possible. It is helpful to remember that most mechanics experience few problems with acne as a direct result of their work. If your son successfully treats his acne with the medication prescribed by his GP, and follows the few simple tips outlined above, it is unlikely that it will cause a problem in his future career.

Costs of NHS prescriptions

I think I am going to have to start paying for my prescriptions soon. Is there any way I can reduce the cost?

Yes. If you are in the minority in the UK who pay for prescriptions, you can lessen the burden by obtaining a prepayment certificate – which is often known as a 'season ticket'. The price is linked to the current cost of prescriptions so can vary but if you have more than around 6 items a quarter or 15 a year it is well worth having. Certificates can cover three months or a full year. Your GP or pharmacist should have details about how to obtain this (from your local primary care organisation) using form FP5.

It is also worth checking whether you are exempt from the prescription charges. Details are given in a leaflet entitled 'Are you entitled to help with health cost?', available from post offices, social security offices or hospitals. In general, you do not have to pay for prescriptions if:

- you are aged 60 or over,

- you are aged under 16,

- you are aged 16, 17 or 18 and in full-time education,

- you (or your adult dependants) are on Income Support, income-based Jobseekers' Allowance, Family Credit or Disability Working Allowance,

- you are pregnant or you have a baby under 12 months old,

- you have certain medical conditions (acne is not one of them),

- you are receiving a War or Ministry of Defence Disablement Pension and need prescribed items because of your disability.

Some of the treatments that are used for acne are available over the counter (without a prescription). Buying them this way is sometimes cheaper than with a prescription. However, do note that it often works the other way, medicines obtained on prescription being cheaper than buying them over the counter. Check with your pharmacist.

Other concerns

My daughter wants to get her ears pierced – should I let her? I am worried that it might make her acne worse.

Please let your daughter get them pierced. It will make no difference to her acne, and will help her feel 'normal' and happier with her appearance. Having earrings will help, as they can help to draw people's attention away from her face.

I am worried that my son is going to do badly in his GCSEs because of his acne. It has really flared up and made him so stressed and unhappy. Is there anything I can do?

As well as making sure he knows you are feeling for him and ensuring that he is still using his treatment, there is one very useful thing you could do. A lot of children have health problems that interfere with their performance in exams, and teachers and examiners are allowed to take this into consideration. Talk to your son's tutor and ask if a letter from your GP would help. If he then gets a lower grade than expected, the medical advice will help in supporting your case. Your GP is entitled to make a small charge for this type of letter.

My son sits in front of his computer for hours playing games. Is this why he has bad acne?

No, there is no connection between computers and acne. Many of his friends will spend just as long as he does in front of a screen and not all of them will have acne. A plus in this connection is that, while he is on the computer, he will be using his hands and won't be tempted to pick or squeeze his spots.

10
Skin-care

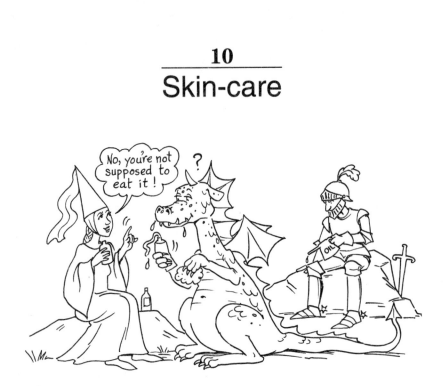

Introduction

Looking after your skin on a daily basis is important for it to feel and look better, but people with skin prone to acne will not be able to cleanse away spots instantly. You should look at skin-care as a complement to acne treatments and be extra careful when selecting the best products for your skin. Too many chemicals, combined with scrubbing or harsh toners, might result in making your acne worse – the very opposite of what you are trying to achieve!

Keep your skin-care routine as simple as possible, especially if you are using prescription creams from your doctor, which may make your skin red or flaky. There follow some helpful tips about skin-care:

- Expensive products are not always the best!

- Look for oil-free or 'non-comedogenic' products that will not clog the pores.

- Look for products that are aimed at oily skin types; these will help reduce surface oil and help keep the skin 'balanced'. (The skin has its own natural level of oiliness, which, if products are too harsh, may be stripped away, resulting in over-dry skin – not very helpful if you have acne, as this will result in the skin working overtime to try to 're-balance' itself.)

- If your skin is dry from prescription creams or lotions, apply plenty of oil-free moisturiser.

- It is OK to wear make-up over any prescription creams or lotions. If your skin gets dry from using these, though, apply the oil-free moisturiser and allow this, together with your acne treatment, 10–15 minutes to be absorbed into the skin before applying foundation or powder. Make sure that your make-up is also oil-free.

- Thoroughly remove all make-up each night.

Skin-care and beauty counters can present an Aladdin's cave of choice. Well-lit displays and attractive assistants can make you feel very intimidated, especially as most of them seem so perfectly made up without a spot or rash in sight! Here is some helpful advice for when you visit a store or counter:

- Don't be intimidated. The counter assistants may look very glamorous, but they have their entire range of make-up to hand. They are meant to look glamorous to attract people to their counter!

- Explain about your skin condition and any treatments that you are using – and don't accept any versions of 'if you change your make-up and buy this product, your acne will go', because it won't . . . *ever*.

- Take a friend with you and don't buy anything until you are sure that your friend agrees with your choice. After all, your friend is more likely to have your best interests at heart, not sales targets.

- Ask to try any products or make-up, or book a make-over so you can see the full results. Then take some time to think about what you really need. If necessary, walk away without buying and let the products stay on your skin all day. Is your skin happy with the products that you have used? Is it more or less greasy than before? You know your skin best. If you are not convinced, don't buy!

- Most staff on skin-care and beauty counters should be happy to let you take home samples before committing yourself. If they don't have sample sizes, take an empty, clean, film cartridge container with you and ask them to put a sample in it for you to try.

- If you are choosing a foundation, it must be a colour match you are going to be really happy with. Don't even think about buying it until you have seen your skin tone in natural daylight. Try it on your face or neck and look at yourself in a mirror (perhaps take one with you). Walk outside and look again. Is it natural enough? Does it look too thick, or too thin, on your skin?

Most acne-type skins are bombarded with products: cleansers, soaps, scrubs, toners, moisturisers, and then acne creams on top. No wonder the skin can't cope. The following routine may be all that is necessary:

- Wash with a pH 5.5 'balanced' soap or soap-free cleanser that you foam up and then wash off. This will prevent the skin's natural oils being stripped away. Rinse with warm (*not* hot) water and gently pat dry.

- Use an exfoliator at least once a week if you feel it is helpful. This is equally suitable for men's and women's skin. Exfoliation helps keep the skin free from a build-up of dead skin cells (which are bad for the acne-prone skin type) as well as smoothing the skin. They usually come as 'masks' and can be left on to work on their own. Rinse off with warm (*not* hot) water

- Apply oil-free moisturiser as often as your skin needs it. Because they do not contain oils, they don't lock in the moisture as much as those containing oil.

- Toners are often alcohol-based and may dry out the skin more than necessary. They will make your skin feel tight and tingly but serve little useful function.

If you visit a beauty salon, remember that most beauticians will have had little, if any, training about acne. It is inevitable that some may suggest you stop taking your treatment and switch to their latest acne-busting products. This is when you should be very cautious and wary. You need to ask yourself why they want you to do this, especially if they have not suggested that you discuss this with your doctor first. Unfortunately, you will often find that the answer lies in sales and not sense. Any reputable clinic will understand that their product range should be used as a complement to any treatment that you are using.

Skin-care and make-up products

I am so confused by skin-care products these days. I want to look after my skin carefully, even though I get regular break-outs, but I seem to end up spending a fortune on products that make claims that don't seem to materialise. What is the best skin-care routine?

Unfortunately, there is no simple answer to this. The skin-care market is a big business, with people spending large amounts a year on these products. There is no one brand that is better than another, especially as our skin's reactions to such products vary so much. In the early 1980s we were told to cleanse, tone and moisturise, but this theory was introduced by a skin-care company that wanted to encourage us to purchase as many products as possible!

Skin-care should be seen as something separate from acne prevention. Although there is no reason why you should not buy these products, keep in mind the fact that no cosmetic product will really be able to help with a medical problem such as active acne – they are simply too 'weak' to have much benefit.

Work out in advance what you are prepared to spend on your new skin-care purchases and stick to it. If you are going to visit a skin-care counter, be prepared to be 'blinded by science' with claims about dermatologist approved, hyper this and hypo that. Often, on closer examination, they can mean very little. The 'bottom line' is: if you need oil-free products, that is what you should ask for. Take a friend with you if necessary, to help you put a brake on huge over-spending!

I want to use a facial wash. Which is the best one?

There is no brand that is particularly better than another. Most of them will describe which skin types they are best suited to. If your problem is greasy, spotty skin, look for products that should be best for you. Remember, though, that these are only skin-care and are not, on their own, always capable of 'curing' your problem. Remember the Acne Support Group's two-month rule: if you don't see a significant improvement after two months, try another product.

My pores are always open and really noticeable. What can I do? I even have tablets from the doctor.

No tablets are going to close any skin pores, even though they may have been given to help reduce the acne problems you are having at present. Once the pores are opened, it is difficult to reduce their size physically, but this is where using good make-up products can help. Open pores happen because the hair follicle has been stretched open with the solid plug that was once a blackhead. These pores will tend to absorb make-up and therefore may still seem quite obvious. You can reduce this by making sure your skin is not too greasy and that your make-up is oil-free. Finish off with a light powder that will 'fix' your foundation, and use the powder as often as necessary. It is likely that over time these open pores may become less obvious.

If you do not use make-up, it is unlikely that you will be able to disguise these pores to any great effect. But make-up is suitable for both men and women, especially some of the ranges available today that provide a skin camouflage – aimed to blend exactly with your skin's own natural colouring without leaving your skin looking as though it is covered in pan stick. There are specialist cosmetic companies that make a range of concealers and foundations suitable for both men and women. Ask your GP to refer you to your local British Red Cross Cosmetic Camouflage or contact them direct through the listing given in the *Useful addresses* appendix.

When my daughter starts isotretinoin (Roaccutane) next week, I would like to really support her by buying her some lovely make-up. What do you recommend?

We suggest that you don't spend your money on make-up just yet. Wait until she has finished her course of treatment (usually four months) and then allow her skin to settle (another month). Then you can take her to a make-up counter in a department store and let them work with her to see what looks best.

While she is taking the isotretinoin treatment, she may be interested in working on enhancing her eyes. They are one of our most revealing features but are often overlooked. Taking attention away from a sore, red face can be easier than you think. If she can practise using make-up to bring her eyes to life and as the main focus of her face, it will help her deal with any acne flare-ups or redness while using isotretinoin. A good beautician will also look at her eyebrow shape and give advice on make-up techniques. In the meantime, perhaps you could give her a pair of earrings.

My friend says that the spots I get on my cheekbone area might be caused by a dirty blusher brush. Is this possible?

This could well be true. How long has it been since you washed your brush? How old is your blusher? Don't forget that make-up products are in direct contact with your skin and, if any of your make-up products has been used for more than 12–18 months, you could be helping to harbour bacteria that may not help with acne-prone skin. Wash any brushes or sponges you use at least once a month, or more if you feel that your skin is particularly prone to being very greasy. Use a detergent and rinse well under a running tap until all colour from your make-up has been washed out and the water is clear. Throw away any unused foundation or powder after one year and buy a new supply. If the only area on your face that is affected by acne is around your cheekbones, you may well find that this change is the answer.

Why is something called non-comedogenic? What exactly does this mean?

'Non-comedogenic' means that it does not contain oils that cause blockages in the hair follicles. In effect, a product that is comedogenic will put a 'lid' on the surface of the skin, making acne worse than before because it forms a trap for the oils building up deep within the hair follicle. With no way of escaping on the surface of the skin, the trapped oils will cause inflammation and bacteria to build up and thus make acne worse.

Moisturising

I use oil-free moisturiser on top of my acne cream but my skin still seems quite dry. First, how long after applying my acne cream should I wait before applying the moisturiser and, second, how often should I apply it?

To answer your first question, it is advisable to allow the acne cream approximately 15 minutes to be absorbed into the skin before applying your moisturiser. This allows it time to penetrate the skin and start working.

Moisturisers are designed to work by preventing water loss from the surface of the skin and trapping it in the outer layer of cells. The greasier or oilier a product is, the longer this effect will last. Because you need to use a light, oil-free moisturiser, this effect will last for only a short time, allowing the skin to dry out again. You can apply the moisturiser as often as you feel that your skin needs it – which can be as often as every hour.

I have acne on my chin, but my cheeks are quite dry. I'm confused about what skin-care products to use.

It's quite amazing how the skin can vary on just one small area of the body – from greasy chin and, just a few centimetres away, dry cheeks. Scan the shelves in your local skin-care counter and you will find a huge range of products claiming to help 'combination' skin.

However, be warned. When you have active acne, even if it is confined to one area of your face, it is not merely a 'greasy skin' problem. The acne needs to be treated (see Chapter 4, *Treatment from your GP*) and these products may be of little real benefit. Using oil-free moisturisers in those dry areas is perfectly adequate and will not help new spots to form in the 'cross-over' area – i.e. where the spotty area meets the dry.

If you are using soap, use a pH 5.5 'balanced' one. (Most cosmetic companies will label their soaps with their pH balance.) This helps to prevent stripping the skin of its natural acid 'mantle' and will therefore reduce further drying. If this does not work, go for a soap substitute bought from your pharmacist.

Camouflage

I am African-Caribbean and have luckily got rid of my spots, but I have terrible dark-coloured, flat marks left around my hairline. I don't know how to cover them up or whether I should use skin bleaching.

This dark skin pigmentation you describe is called *post-acne pigmentation*. It is a result of your skin type, which is more likely to lay down more melanin than, say, Caucasian skin. These marks are very likely to fade of their own accord in time. In the meantime, there are some excellent camouflage creams available from some UK companies that have designed a range of creams to match *any* skin colour.

The British Red Cross Camouflage Service is free, and you should ask your doctor for a referral to it. It is usually based in the dermatology clinic of the local hospital. There may be a waiting list, but the results can be amazing.

The way camouflage works is to disguise any flat pigmentation or scars, blending in naturally with your natural skin tone. The British Red Cross cosmetic camouflage experts often show you how to apply it, in effect giving you a free individual lesson, to help build your confidence. You will also be shown how to use their 'fixing' powder, which keeps the creams on for up to three days. These are just as suitable for men as they are for women.

The skin bleaching you asked about should be avoided, as it can have long-term consequences and possibly make the affected skin permanently lighter. Giving your skin a chance to heal and disguising it in the meantime is probably the best option but, if you are very keen to try something now, talk to your GP. A combination of some of the creams that are used to treat acne can help extra pigmentation. Azelaic acid and a retinoid cream are a popular combination.

Other products

**I keep hearing about tea tree oil products, but I don't
know what percentage of tea tree oil is actually in these
products. I imagine that the less there is, the less
effective it will be. What is your advice?**

Tea tree oil is one of the few essential oils that can be applied
direct to the skin, but it can be very drying, so go sparingly. It
doesn't really matter how much tea tree oil the product contains,
it's whether it works that counts. As ordinary skin-care, it may be
very helpful, but if you want treat acne, remember the two-month
rule (see Chapter 4, *Treatment from your GP*); move on to
another treatment if you are not happy with the results after two
months.

**My main problem is blackheads around my nose, which are
awful. I have seen these silver 'comedone spoons' that are
supposed to help squeeze them out. Do you recommend
these or are they just a gimmick?**

The comedone spoons you mention are designed to help squeeze
the thick, wiggly type of pus from blackheads – in effect, clearing
them out. It is not a matter of whether they are good or bad, it is
down to each individual's preference. However, there are dangers
that the spoon may either not fully extract the contents or will
leave a bright red round mark where it has had to be pressed so
hard onto the skin – thus leaving you with something potentially
more obvious! The answer is to *not* use the spoon ten minutes
before you go out, as the skin will need time to calm down. If you
use a hot compress on your skin before the spoon, this will make
it much easier.

Other ways of extracting blackheads include the facial strips
that are readily available from pharmacies/chemist shops. These
act like glue and literally stick to the top of the blackheads and
'strips' them off. Once again, there are a few good reasons why
you shouldn't use these, including a potential to irritate the skin

in between the blackheads. If, however, you have a constant ongoing problem with blackheads and whiteheads (see Chapter 1, *What is acne?*), you may find a prescription cream containing a retinoid more helpful; this will loosen the plug while helping to reduce inflammation. The cream won't be an instant cure, but can help with more persistent blackheads.

I have regular facial saunas, but I have now heard these aren't recommended to help with acne. This is very confusing, and I must admit I quite like the sauna, as my face feels really refreshed afterwards.

Experts tend to agree that saunas only do half a job in helping the skin. The theory is that they open the pores of the face, allowing the trapped 'debris' to be released. Although saunas will open the skin pores, it is not complete enough for clogged-up pores to just 'release' themselves on their own. Once the skin has cooled, sweat is still trapped in the follicle, together with the sebum and dead skin cells (the main culprits in acne), and this combination could actually make matters worse. If you use a sauna too regularly, you may find that the skin starts to 'break out', as it finds it hard to keep up with such direct heat, open pores and sweat. Use clean cotton pads soaked in a gentle cleanser to help remove any excess sweat or grease once you have used a sauna.

It is fair to say that some people find it relaxing and refreshing to use a sauna – whether facial or full – but our advice is to stay away from them if you have a problem with acne eruptions. Any sort of steamy environment is no good for acne-prone skin.

My GP has suggested that I try an exfoliant. How do exfoliants work and how often should I use them?

Some GPs are happy to prescribe a type of exfoliant that helps to remove some of the dead skin cells that may be helping to block the surface of the skin pores. However, there is a huge range of other exfoliants available that you can buy off the shelf. They can play a valuable role in helping your skin feel and look smoother but will not replace any acne treatment. Don't be tempted to use them more than once a week – your skin will know what it is happy to tolerate.

My pharmacist has suggested a wash containing salicylic acid. This sounds a bit harsh. Would it help?

Salicylic acid is related to aspirin and used to be popular as a treatment before retinoids came along. It is quite irritant when left on the skin but there are washes available that you apply to the skin and then wash off. Some people find them helpful and believe that they help reduce the numbers of comedones. This is because they can clear some of the dead skin in the pores and keep them clear. There is no hard evidence that they are any better than ordinary soap and water but they are safe to try.

Can I still use sunscreen even though I have acne?

Yes, you can. It is very important to protect your skin from the damaging effects of UV light and its potential to worsen your acne. You will still get a tan despite the sunscreen.

Think of sunscreens in the same way that you do moisturisers and make-up products. Go for light ones that are non-comedogenic and wait 15 minutes after applying your acne treatment before smoothing on the sunscreen. Don't rub it in vigorously, as this could irritate your skin and leave you with too thin a layer to protect you.

Some topical treatments and antibiotic tablets can make you more sensitive to the sun – check with your GP or pharmacist and read the information leaflets with the medication.

11
Research and future treatments

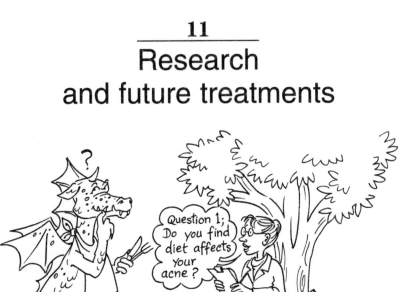

Introduction

Acne has been around as long as man can remember – it comes from the Greek word 'akme', which means pimple – but it is only in the last 25 years that we have seen a variety of effective treatments becoming available. It's amazing to think that your grandparents may have had to endure the misery of spots with no medical help except for smelly sulphur creams or, in more severe cases, x-ray treatment. Even people now in their 50s or 60s would have had no treatment options other than one type of antibiotic tablet. Doctors are now able to prescribe their patients a combination of over 100 treatments. No one yet has tried every treatment available! As technology advances, we are seeing the introduction of new, novel ways of treating acne, such as light therapy or laser technology. Most of these have been developed in the USA, a country with an estimated 300 million people with acne.

Throughout this book you will have noticed some admissions that there is still a lot we do not fully understand about acne. We know what happens in the skin and that sensitivity to hormones plays an important role but why and how the whole process starts is still unclear. Over the years our knowledge has grown and, with it, the treatment regimens have become more effective. Doctors used to advise squeezing and pinching the skin vigorously every day to express all the sebum from the pores but we now know that these, along with x-rays and other options, actually do more harm than good. Treatment regimens are still not ideal, as many have side-effects and can be awkward to fit into normal life.

Research is needed into complementary approaches to treatment but large, properly set up research studies are very costly. Nevertheless, it is only positive results from these types of studies that allow new treatments to gain wider acceptance and even become available on the NHS.

Where we are now

Before we look for new treatments, however, it would be sensible to make the most of what we have. Time and again, the questions we are asked reflect the lack of interest that some health professionals have in treating acne and in understanding the huge impact it can have on our quality of life. There is a real and urgent need to put more emphasis on skin disease in the training programmes for doctors, nurses and pharmacists. The average GP's workload contains 10–15 per cent of consultations to do with the skin yet there is no formal requirement to study skin disease in GP training. Many GPs will attend courses once they are in a practice and some become very expert indeed but this is no help if your own GP knows very little about your acne.

If acne is so treatable, why are there still millions of people who have it, even with the loads of treatments available?

We are all slightly different from one another, and acne treatments that are very effective for one person might not work for another. This is the case for a lot of treatments designed to help skin diseases. Therefore, for some people, finding an effective treatment may take a lot of time and effort. Also, remembering to apply creams daily and/or take tablets at certain times can interfere with everyday life. It is fair to say that you have to be very determined to stick at any treatment to get the best results. So it is not always a matter of the treatment itself failing but our willingness to stick to it properly and completely. Members of the Acne Support Group report that, on average, they have tried over six different types of treatment, and they still may not have found what they consider to be a 'totally effective' treatment.

My friend's GP seems to be a bit of an expert in acne. Why can't I go to see him?

It might be possible to change doctors but this depends on whether you live in that GP's catchment area and whether he has any room on his list to take you on as well. GPs look after an average of just under 2000 patients each, and increasing these numbers could create an impossible rise in workload.

In the near future you might be able to see this GP if he really does have a special interest and extra training. He could then work some of the time as a specialist GP – either at his practice or at a separate clinic – at a kind of intermediate point between GP and hospital care. Patients who needed some extra help but not the full hospital service would see the specialist GP, who could suggest the best kind of treatment for their own GP to pre-scribe. This is likely to happen for a range of medical specialities, and dermatology will certainly be one of them. You should be able to find out more from your local primary care organisation.

In the meantime, if your GP works in a group that has practice nurses, you may find that one of them has a special interest in skin problems.

Research for new treatments

I seem to have come to a dead end with the treatments I can try. Are there going to be any new drugs to treat acne?

This is a common question from anyone with a long-term medical problem. Research is going on into new types of drug that could switch off sebum production and into drugs that like an oily envi-ronment so will be taken up into the pores to concentrate their action where the problem is. These drugs will act to decrease inflammation and to kill the *P. acnes* bacteria.

Researchers are also looking at new topical antibiotics to kill the resistant bacteria. A lot of the damage in acne is done by the body's own defence reaction from the immune system. If this could be switched off locally, it would make a great difference to the inflammation and future scarring. It would not be safe to try to switch off the whole of the immune system, as that would lead to serious problems in fighting off other illnesses and infections. All drugs take a long time to evolve from an idea, through devel-opment and then the trials and red tape necessary to license them for use. For most companies it can take many years to develop a treatment and make it available for doctors to pre-scribe. It may be the next generation that benefits from new treatments developed with the hope of making acne therapy more effective. But we might yet see our dream of 'curing' acne come true.

Is there any acne research that I could help with?

This depends to some extent on how bad your acne is and where you live. But research is continuing and there may be different research projects you could help with. If you are keen, check with the Acne Support Group and contact your local hospital's dermatology department, explaining that you'd be interested in getting involved in research projects.

I would like to help research but don't want to be a human guinea-pig for new drugs. Can I still help?

Yes, you can. Much of the research that is needed will not involve new drugs. The other areas of research that might appeal to you are:

- **Safety studies** on existing treatments, such as isotretinoin, to reduce side-effects.

- **Predictive studies** that try to find the reasons why some people don't get acne.

- **Psychological studies** that look at the effect of acne on quality of life and try to see if certain personality types are more likely to get acne.

- **Research** into complementary medicines and treatments.

The results obtained from these types of studies often give experts information that will help them to change the way treatments are offered and at what stage they may be offered, and to expand the current choices of acne therapies a doctor can offer. The Acne Support Group often invites its members to take part in trials or research, giving people with acne a chance to feel more involved or to influence the future of acne treatments.

Surely, in this new millennium, we will be able to find the ultimate cure for acne? I think we should get scientists to look at genes and then help us to eradicate it once and for all. Do you agree?

Gene therapy has been talked about for years as the ultimate treatment but we are a long way away from achieving it. The best hope is to identify the genes involved in a disease and then gain more understanding of what each gene does and what goes wrong in disease. This will help in the development of drugs that will be more targeted to the malfunction with fewer side-effects. But we must be careful about trying to breed acne-free humans – who knows what good effects of some of those genes would be lost forever.

Glossary

Terms in *italic* in the definitions are also defined in this Glossary.

abscess a swelling from a localised collection of pus, kept separate by a surrounding wall of damaged and inflamed tissue

acute short-lasting. In medical terms, this usually means lasting for days rather than weeks or months. (*See also* chronic)

adrenal glands important glands in the body that produce a number of *hormones* to control the body systems. Cortisol and cortisone are two very important examples, and adrenaline is another.

allergy to have an allergy means that your body over-reacts to something in a harmful way when you come into contact with it. If you have an allergy to grass pollen you will have streaming eyes and nose and sneezing if you come into contact with it (hay-fever). Someone who is not allergic to grass pollen will not even notice when they have come into contact with it.

androgens *hormones* that stimulate *sebaceous glands* and have an effect on hair growth in addition to other effects on the body. Present in both males and females but at higher levels in males

anecdotal evidence reports from people about their experience of *triggers*, treatment, etc. – rather than scientific evidence obtained from strictly regulated tests

antibody a special kind of blood protein made in response to a particular *antigen*, which is designed to attack the antigen

antigen any substance that the body regards as foreign or potentially dangerous

atrophy wasting away of a body tissue. With skin this means thinning and loss of strength

biopsy the process of obtaining a sample of tissue for examination under a microscope

blackhead an open, non-inflamed *comedone*

chronic in strictly medical terms, chronic means long-lasting or persistent. Many people use the word 'chronic' incorrectly to mean severe or extreme. (*See also* acute)

closed comedone (whitehead) a *comedone* with a white centre due to closure of the opening of the *sebaceous gland*

comedogenic likely to cause *comedones*

comedone a typical acne *lesion* resulting from blockage in the opening of the *sebaceous gland*

corticosteroids *see* steroids

cyst a swelling filled with fluid or semi-solid matter

dermatology the medical speciality concerned with the diagnosis and treatment of skin disease

dermis the deep layer of the skin

diagnostic something that occurs so often in a disease that you don't need any other clues to know what the disease is

distribution the pattern of a disease on the skin; for example, all over, on the forehead, on the back, etc.

eczema a red, itchy inflammation of the skin, sometimes with blisters and weeping

emollient an agent that soothes and softens the skin; also known as a moisturiser

epidermis the outer layer of the skin

exfoliator helps to remove dead cells from the skin surface

genes units of inheritance that make up an individual's characteristics. Half are inherited from each parent

genetic to do with *genes*

hormone a substance that is produced in a gland in one part of the body and is carried in the bloodstream to work in other parts of the body

immune system the body's defence system against outside 'attackers' whether they are infections, injuries or agents that are recognised as 'foreign'. The immune system fights off infection and produces *antibodies* that will protect against future attack

immunity resistance to specific disease(s) because of *antibodies* produced by the body's *immune system*

immunosuppressive a drug that reduces the body's resistance to infection and other foreign bodies by suppressing the immune reaction. (*See also* immune system)

incidence the number of new cases of an illness arising in a population over a given time

inflammation the reaction of the body to an injury, infection or disease. Generally, it will protect the body against the spread of injury or infection, but may become *chronic*, when it tends to damage the body rather than protect it

keloid an abnormal overgrowth of scar tissue

keratinocytes types of cells that make up over 95 per cent of the *epidermis*, or outer layer of the skin

lesion an abnormal area of tissue

lipids oily substances including fats, oils and waxes. Some can be irritating to the skin

lymphocytes white blood cells that are involved in *immunity*

macule a small flat area of skin of a different colour from normal

mechanical a direct effect on the skin from physical pressure, friction or trauma

microcomedone the first stage of *comedone* formation before anything can be seen on the skin

milia a small, white lump in the skin

moisturiser *see* emollient

natural history the normal course of a disease, the way it develops over time

nodule the most severe type of acne *lesion*. A large, deep, painful lump, often containing pus. Difficult to distinguish from a *cyst* but harder and deeper in the skin

non-comedogenic unlikely to cause *comedones*

papular a pattern of rash that consists of small raised spots on the skin less than 5mm in diameter (papules)

photosensitiser any agent, *topical* or *systemic*, that acts to increase the sensitivity of the skin to light

phototherapy treatment with light – usually ultraviolet (UV) light

polycystic containing a large number of *cysts*

pomade a hair 'treatment' containing oils or greases

***Propionibacterium acnes* (*P. acnes*)** a bacterium that is normally present on the skin but which will multiply rapidly in blocked pores where *sebum* is trapped

psychologist a specialist who studies behaviour and its related mental processes

puberty the time of life when a child starts maturing physically into an adult. It is accompanied by an increase in the production of *hormones*

pus a thick yellow–green fluid containing white cells, dead and living bacteria and other dead cells associated with infection and inflammation

pustules a *pus*-containing swelling arising out of an inflamed *comedone*

rosacea a *chronic* inflammatory skin disease affecting the face

sebaceous glands glands in the skin that produce an oily substance – *sebum*

seborrhoeic related to excessive secretion of *sebum*. (*See also* sebaceous glands)

sebum the oily substance produced by the *sebaceous glands* and passed on to the skin surface through small ducts. It provides a thin layer on the skin, helping to prevent water loss

steroids a particular group of chemicals, which includes very important *hormones*, produced naturally by the body, and also many drugs used for a wide range of medical purposes. In medical treatment the subgroup of steroids with which we are concerned is the corticosteroids. Very often this term is shortened to 'steroids', causing people to confuse their treatments with the anabolic steroids used for body building

subcutaneous beneath the skin

systemic this term is used for a drug given by mouth or injection that affects the whole body

teratogenic something that damages an unborn child

topical a term used to describe drugs that are applied to the skin rather than being taken internally

triggers factors that may bring on acne but do not actually cause it

white blood cells parts of the blood and *immune system* that help fight off infections

whitehead a closed *comedone*

Appendix 1
Useful Addresses

Please note that website addresses change quite frequently and quickly become out of date.

Useful organisations

Acne Support Group
PO Box 9
Newquay TR9 6WG
Tel: 0870 870 2263
Website: www.stopspots.org
A registered charity that provides independent advice and support for anyone affected by acne or rosacea. Telephone for a free factsheet. Membership gives access to a range of information covering all aspects of acne.

Associate Parliamentary Group on Skin
3/19 Holmbush Road
London SW15 3LE
Tel: 020 8246 6428
Fax: 020 8789 0795
An all-party group specialising in skin, established in 1993 to raise awareness in Parliament of skin disease. Individual membership is available.

British Association of Dermatologists/British Dermatological Nursing Group
19 Fitzroy Square
London W1T 6EH
Tel: 020 7383 0266
Fax: 020 7388 5263
Website: www.bad.org.uk
Professional organisations representing doctors and nurses who have an interest in and/or work directly in dermatology. Among other things they provide patient-information leaflets about various skin disorders. They can also supply a list of NHS dermatologists in your area.

British Association of Aesthetic Plastic Surgeons
Royal College of Surgeons
35–43 Lincoln's Inn Fields
London WC2A 3PE
Tel: 020 7430 1840
Advice line: 020 7405 2234
Website: www.baaps.org.uk
Information service on scars and keloids, lasers and plastic surgery; also provides list of NHS and private surgeons. Please send s.a.e.

British Association of Skin Camouflage
c/o Resources for Business
South Park Road
Macclesfield SK11 6SH
Tel: 01625 267880
Fax: 01625 267879
Website: www.skin-camouflage.net
A network of NHS and private practitioners trained in remedial camouflage techniques for skin conditions and disfiguring injuries. Can refer to nearest practitioner.

British Complementary Medicine Association
PO Box 5122
Bournemouth BH8 0WG
Tel: 0845 345 5977
Fax: 0845 345 5978
Website: www.bcma.co.uk
Multi-therapy umbrella body representing organisations, clinics, colleges and independent schools, and acting as the voice of complementary medicine.

British Red Cross
9 Grosvenor Crescent
London SW1X 7EJ
Tel: 020 7201 5173
Fax: 020 7235 7447
Website: www.redcross.org.uk
For free advice and information
on cosmetic camouflage to cover
up any skin condition,
including acne scarring. Refers
you to local branches.

Changing Faces
1 & 2 Junction Mews
London W2 1PN
Tel: 020 7706 4232
Fax: 020 7706 4234
Website:
www.changingfaces.co.uk
A charity that helps people
facially disfigured in any way to
express themselves with more
confidence, and combats many of
their anxieties and negative
feelings.

ChildLine
Studd Street
London N1 0QW
Tel: 020 7239 1000
Fax: 020 7239 1001
Childline: 0800 1111
Website: www.childline.org.uk
Confidential, free helpline UK-
wide for children and young
people who are in trouble or
danger. Offers counselling and
referral to appropriate agencies.
Outreach visits to school and
information sheets.

Disfigurement Guidance
Centre
PO Box 7
Cupar
Fife KY15 4PF
Tel: 01337 870281
Fax: 01337 870310
Website:
www.skinlaserdirectory.org.uk
Produces annual directory that
lists where skin laser treatment
is carried out, whether NHS or
private; contains articles on
latest research and is freely
available to health professionals
or can be purchased for £5.
Cannot deal with phone
enquiries, so please send s.a.e.

Eating Disorders Association
1st floor,
103 Prince of Wales Road
Norwich
Norfolk NR1 1DW
Tel: 0870 770 3256
Fax: 01603 664 915
Helpline: 0845 634 1414 (Mon–Fri
9a.m.–6.30p.m.)
Youth Helpline: 0845 634 7656
(Mon–Fri 4–6p.m.)
Website: www.edauk.com
Offers information, help and
support to anyone affected by
eating disorders – anorexia and
bulimia nervosa.

Institute for Complementary
Medicine
PO Box 194
London SE16 1QZ
Tel: 020 7237 5165 (weekdays
10a.m.–2p.m.)
Fax: 020 7237 5175
Website: icmedicine.co.uk
Umbrella group for
complementary medicine
organisations. Offers informed,
safe advice to public, has
register of British practitioners
and refers to accredited training
courses. (Please send self-
addressed envelope and two 2nd
class stamps.)

MIND
15–19 Broadway
London E15 4BQ
Tel: 020 8519 2122
Fax: 020 8522 1725
Website: www.mind.org.uk
MIND Infoline: 0845 766 0163
Publications order line: 020 8221
9666
Mental health organisation
working for a better life for
everyone experiencing mental
distress. Has information and
offers support via local branches.

NHS Direct (Health
Information Service)
0845 4647
Information about the NHS,
including services available in
your area. They also have details
about patient support groups,
conditions and possible
treatment.

Obsessive Action
Aberdeen Centre
22–24 Highbury Grove
London N5 2EA
Tel: 020 7226 4545
Helpline: 020 7226 4000
Fax: 020 7228 0828
Website: www.obsessive-
action.demon.co.uk
Offers advice on where to go to
get help. Has free written
information and sells videos and
CDs.

Outlook Disfigurement Support Unit
Ward 22
Frenchay Hospital
Bristol BS16 1LE
Tel: 0117 975 3992 ext 3891
For help dealing with the scarring resulting from acne and other skin disorders. NHS referral only.

Primary Care Dermatology Society
PO Box 6
Princes Risborough HP7 9XD
Tel: 01844 276271
Fax: 01844 342278
An organisation made up of GPs who have a special interest in dermatology.

Skin Care Campaign
Hill House
Highgate Hill
London N19 5NA
Website:
www.skincarecampaign.org
An alliance of patient groups, health professionals and other organisations concerned with skin care. It campaigns for a better deal for people with a wide variety of skin problems. Very limited resources prevent them from taking enquiries from the general public but they have a website.

Skinship
Plascow Cottage
Kirkgunzeon
Dumfries DG2 8JT
Helpline: 01387 760 567
Website:
www.ukselfhelp.info/skinship
Provides information for people with any skin disorder, the aim being to 'ease the pain and end the shame'.

Skin Treatment and Research Trust (START)
Chelsea and Westminster Hospital
369 Fulham Road
London SW10 9NH
Tel: 020 8746 8174
Fax: 020 8746 8887
Email: gail-start@email.com
Primarily a laboratory research establishment, not an information service, but they may be able to give information about specific research questions. They also raise funds for research into skin disease.

Useful websites for teenagers

www.bullying.co.uk
The website of Bullying Online, a registered charity, it gives all sorts of information and advice about coping with bullying

www.bullying.org
A Canadian website about bullying, with contributions from around the world

www.mykindaplace.com
An online magazine, updated daily, that includes a section on health

Appendix 2
Useful Publications

Useful publications for people with acne

Does the Way You Look Really Matter? obtainable from the
  Disfigurement Guidance Centre (address in Appendix 1)
  1 899219 02 1
Solving Skin Problems, by Ricki Ostrov, published by Marshall
  Editions, London (1999) 1 84028102 2
Spots and Other Skin Problems, by Anita Naik, published by
  Knight Publishing, London (2000) 0 34075737 X
The Good Skin Doctor, by Anne Lovell and Tony Chu, published
  by HarperCollins, London (1999) 0 7 2253675 5

Useful publications for healthcare professionals

ABC of Dermatology, 2nd edition, edited by P K Buxton,
  published by BMJ books, London (1999) 0 72791404 9
Acne: diagnosis and management, by J Strauss, W Cunliffe,
  H Gollnick and A Lucky, published by Martin Dunitz, London
  (2000) 1 8531 7206 5
Practical Problems in Dermatology, by Ronald Marks,
  published by Martin Dunitz, London (1996) 1 8531 7050 X

Index